Endoscopy and Biopsy in Gastroenterology

Technique and Indications

Edited by
P. Frühmorgen and M. Classen

Translated by
H. V. Ammon and K. H. Soergel

With contributions by
K. Arnold M. Classen K. Elster P. Frühmorgen
H. Henning R. Hohner H. Koch H. Lindner†
D. Look B. C. Manegold G. Menghini
Chr. Romfeld W. Rösch L. Wannagat
S. Weidenhiller W. Wenz

With a Foreword by L. Demling

108 illustrations

Springer-Verlag
Berlin Heidelberg New York

PD Dr. Peter Frühmorgen
Medizinische Universitätsklinik
Krankenhausstraße 12
8520 Erlangen
Federal Republic of Germany

Prof. Dr. Meinhard Classen
Leiter der Abteilung für Gastroenterologie
Zentrum der Inneren Medizin
Johann Wolfgang Goethe Universität
Theodor Stern Kai 7
6000 Frankfurt/Main 70
Federal Republic of Germany

Prof. Helmut V. Ammon, M.D.
The Medical College of Wisconsin
Wood Veterans Administration Center
Milwaukee, Wisconsin 53193
U.S.A.

Prof. Konrad H. Soergel, M.D.
The Medical College of Wisconsin
Milwaukee County General Hospital
8700 West Wisconsin Avenue
Milwaukee, Wisconsin 53226
U.S.A.

Translated from *Endoskopie und Biopsie in der Gastroenterologie*, Second Edition, Revised, Springer-Verlag, 1979.

Library of Congress Cataloging in Publication Data

Frühmorgen, Peter, 1940-
Endoscopy and biopsy in gastroenterology.

Translation of Endoskopie und Biopsie in der Gastroenterologie.
Includes bibliographies and index.
1. Gastroenterology. 2. Endoscope and Endoscopy.
3. Digestive organs—Biopsy.
I. Classen, M., joint author. II. Arnold, Konrad. III. Title.
RC804.E6F7813 616.3'07'54 79-19746

9 8 7 6 5 4 3 2 1

ISBN-13:978-3-540-09645-0 e-ISBN-13:978-3-642-67429-7
DOI: 10.1007/978-3-642-67429-7

Foreword

Gastroenterologic endoscopy has made important progress in the past decade. New techniques and ideas have given it new life. The end of this evolution is not yet in sight. Fully flexible fiberoptic instruments have eliminated all blank areas from the map of the gastrointestinal tract. Retrograde visualization of the pancreatic and biliary system has been achieved in conjunction with radiologic methods. Operative endoscopy has developed beyond the removal of foreign bodies, to a stage where laparotomy can be avoided in a number of situations. Hemostasis by laser coagulation and crushing of concrements by ultrasound and electric energy have reached the threshold of clinical applicability. With all these spectacular developments, however, it is important to maintain a firm grasp of the fundamentals of endoscopy. This is the basis of day-to-day success and includes knowledge of the proper indications, the ability to manage complications, familiarity with the technical properties of the instruments, their skillful handling, and experience in organizing an endoscopy section. Endoscopists, particularly members of the Erlangen group, have undertaken the task of charting these fundamentals and of compiling them into a working manual for those already practicing endoscopy or intending to do so. They have been supported in this effort by colleagues from other parts of the Federal Republic of Germany and from Italy. If it is true that one should not lose sight of the bumpy road ahead while gazing at the stars, then this booklet meets this need and I predict its success.

L. Demling

Introduction

Gastrointestinal diagnostic procedures are designed to yield prompt morphologic confirmation of the preliminary clinical and radiologic diagnosis. No diagnostic approach is better suited to this purpose than endoscopic examination of hollow viscera with preoperative removal of tissue particles from the accessible organs.

The development of appropriate instruments and of practical, effective, and economical methods is the result of close cooperation between biomedical technologists, pathologists, and endoscopists.

Some endoscopic procedures that only a few years ago were considered impossible or were limited to a few gastrointestinal centers, today are considered routine and of high diagnostic efficacy. Even at the present stage, the full potential of this approach has not yet been realized.

The authors of this pocketbook thought it timely to make current knowledge and experience accessible to all those who would like to learn and practice methods of gastrointestinal endoscopy and biopsy. A solid basis of technical skills is necessary to keep complications at a minimum; similarly, knowledge of the place of endoscopy within the framework of all diagostic and therapeutic options is a prerequisite for its appropriate application.

Those contributors who originated, or who helped originate, certain diagnostic methods were encouraged to present their personal experiences and, occasionally, their biases. A comprehensive review of the literature was not intended. Rather, highly experienced specialists were asked to express their own opinions.

The brief, sometimes note-like style of the text allowed condensation of the voluminous material into a pocketbook. The emphasis on practical aspects and line drawings is a didactic device to facilitate learning of the techniques; selected literature references should stimulate further and more extensive study. The uniform format of the chapters is intended to allow quick orientation and to encourage the use of this book as a reference manual. The general section is intended equally for the physician and the technical and nursing personnel, while the detailed description of endoscopic procedures is combined in a special section.

We would like to thank our co-authors for their willingness to adapt a description of their special topics to these considerations. A special debt is owed Professor Soergel and Professor Ammon for their excellent translation and cooperation which made it possible to present this edition.

P. Frühmorgen and M. Classen

Erlangen and Frankfurt, Spring 1980

Contents

Contributors

ARNOLD, K., Priv.-Doz. Dr.; Deutsche Klinik für Diagnostik, Aukamm-Allee 33, 6200 Wiesbaden, Federal Republic of Germany.

CLASSEN, M., Prof. Dr.; Leiter der Abteilung für Gastroenterologie, Zentrum der Inneren Medizin, Johann Wolfgang Goethe Universität Frankfurt, Theodor Stern Kai 7, 6000 Frankfurt/Main 70, Federal Republic of Germany.

ELSTER, K., Prof. Dr.; Leiter des Pathologischen Institutes der Städt. Krankenanstalten, Kulmbacher Straße 23, 8580 Bayreuth, Federal Republic of Germany.

FRÜHMORGEN, P., Priv.-Doz. Dr.; Medizinische Universitätsklinik, Krankenhausstraße 12, 8520 Erlangen, Federal Republic of Germany.

HENNING, H., Priv.-Doz. Dr.; Leiter der Klinik Föhrenkamp der Bundesversicherungsanstalt f. Angestellte, Birkenweg 24, 2410 Mölln, Federal Republic of Germany.

HOHNER, R., Schwester; Abteilung für Gastroenterologie, Zentrum der Inneren Medizin, Johann Wolfgang Goethe Universität Frankfurt, Theodor Stern Kai 7, 6000 Frankfurt/Main 70, Federal Republic of Germany.

KOCH, H., Prof. Dr.; Chefarzt der Gastroenterologischen Abteilung der Städt. Krankenanstalten, Robert Koch Str. 1, 8720 Schweinfurt, Federal Republic of Germany.

LINDNER, H., Prof. Dr.†; formerly Chefarzt der Medizinischen Abteilung des DRK-Krankenhauses, Beim Schlump 84, 2000 Hamburg 13, Federal Republic of Germany.

LOOK, D., Dr.; Leitender Arzt der Klinik Hellbachtal der BFA, Sebastian Kneipp Straße, 2410 Mölln, Federal Republic of Germany.

MANEGOLD, B.C., Priv.-Doz. Dr.; Chirurgische Klinik der Fakultät für Klinische Medizin Mannheim der Universität Heidelberg, Postfach 23, 6800 Mannheim 1, Federal Republic of Germany.

MENGHINI, G., Prof. Dr.; Via Bontempi 40-C.P. 336, I-06100, Perugia, Italy.

ROMFELD, Chr., Schwester; Abteilung für Gastroenterologie, Zentrum der Inneren Medizin, Johann Wolfgang Goethe Universität Frankfurt, Theodor Stern Kai 7, 6000 Frankfurt/Main 70, Federal Republic of Germany.

RÖSCH, W., Priv.-Doz. Dr.; Medizinische Universitätsklinik, Krankenhausstraße 12, 8520 Erlangen, Federal Republic of Germany.

WANNAGAT, L., Prof. Dr.; Ärztlicher Leiter der Bad Mergentheimer Leberklinik, Lothar-Daiker-Straße, 6990 Bad Mergentheim, Federal Republic of Germany.

WEIDENHILLER, S., Dr.; Frauenbergl 2, 8400 Regensburg, Federal Republic of Germany.

WENZ, W., Prof. Dr.; Direktor des Institutes für Röntgendiagnostik der Universität Freiburg, Hugstetter Straße 55, 7800 Freiburg, Federal Republic of Germany.

1

General Section

1.1

Organization of an Endoscopy Service

P. FRÜHMORGEN

1.1.1 Design and Equipment of the Endoscopy Suite

The design and equipment of a modern endoscopy suite are less determined by technological developments and the desires of the endoscopist than by the availability of space and financial resources. This fact will be taken into consideration as far as possible by describing minimal as well as optimal working conditions.

A well functioning, modern endoscopy suite will have to meet the following requirements:

a) Examining rooms that can easily be cleaned, preferably tiled, with the potential for aseptic working conditions (Fig. 1). The rooms should be air-conditioned with exhaust to the outside and have insulated floors if general anesthesia and electrosurgical procedures are to be performed. Fluoroscopy and roentgenographic documentation of findings during endoscopic retrograde cholangiopancreatography, papillotomy, enteroscopy, and colonoscopy should be possible (Fig. 8).
b) Facilities for cleaning, sterilization, and storage of the instruments (Figs. 2–4).
c) Waiting room for ambulatory and inpatients (Fig. 5).
d) Record storage room (written reports, photographs, movies, and X rays) (Figs. 6 and 7).
e) Appropriate work and office areas for physicians and nursing personnel.
f) Secretary's office; secretarial functions can, of course, also be performed in another area of the clinic.

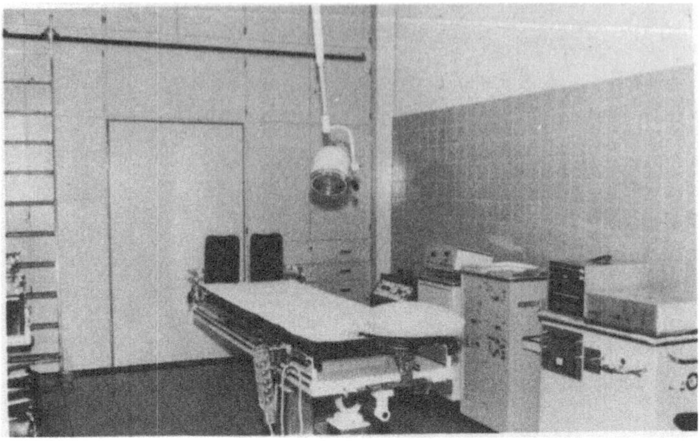

Fig. 1. Partially tiled endoscopy room with wall cabinet and endoscopy table with adjustable height and tilt (Maquet).

Number and size of the rooms required depend upon the nature and volume of the endoscopic procedures. These rooms should never be assigned any additional function. Frequently, one will have to convert rooms already available that had been designed for different purposes. This requires adjustment of the plans for remodeling to the dictates of the local situation. Therefore, we can only give suggestions, rather than rules which are universally applicable.

The anticipated volume of procedures and the level of training of the

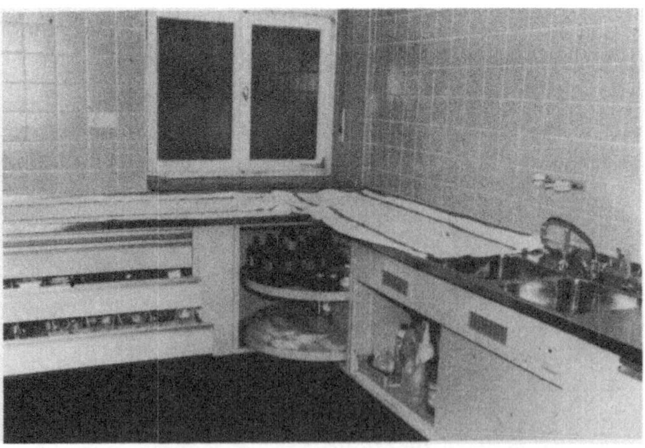

Fig. 2. Working area for cleaning and maintenance of the instruments.

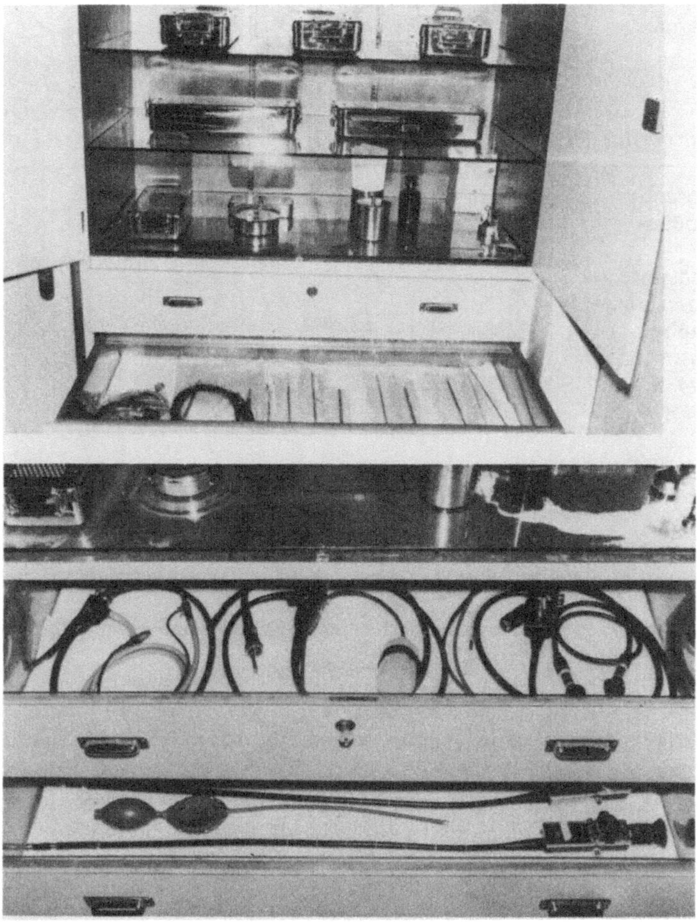

Figs. 3 and 4. Wall cabinets and drawers for storage of instruments.

endoscopists should determine which of the various endoscopic techniques are to be performed. This will permit economical utilization of the rooms and available equipment (Table 1).

An endoscopy room should provide for examination of the patients without distractions, as well as for instrument maintenance and storage, and documentation of the endoscopic findings. This can be accomplished in a single room, although this arrangement may not be optimal. In the face of such physical limitations, however, one can only plan on performing a few simple endoscopic procedures, and particular attention must be paid to problems of asepsis and of sterile conditions during laparoscopy.

Table 1. Gastrointestinal endoscopy in office practice, community hospitals, and medical centers.

Endoscopic procedure	*General practitioner/ internist*	*Hospital*	*Medical (gastroenterology) center*
Proctosigmoidoscopy	+	+	+
Esophagogastroduodenoscopy[a]	−	+	+
Postbulbar duodenoscopy[a]	−	+	+
Retrograde pancreatico-cholangiography	−	+	+
Jejunoileoscopy (enteroscopy)	−	−	+
Partial colonoscopy[a]	−	+	+
Colonoscopy[a]	−	+	+
Ileoscopy	−	−	+
Therapeutic endoscopy[a]	−	+	+
Laparoscopy	−	+	+

Source: Classen M et al.: Gastrointestinale Endoskopie. Versuch einer Bewertung. Internist (Berlin *14*, 245 (1973).

[a] These procedures are occasionally also performed by gastroenterologists in private practice.

The basic equipment of a single endoscopy room includes hand-washing facilities, an examining table with adjustable height and tilt for laparoscopy, an X-ray viewbox, a movable instrument table with lower shelf, a sink for instrument cleaning, a locked cabinet with shelves for the

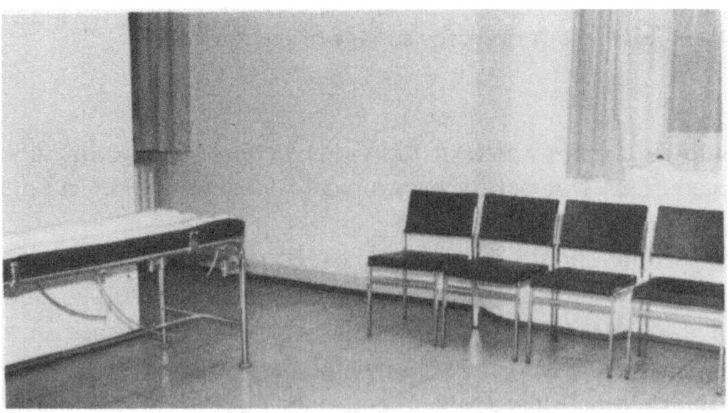

Fig. 5. Waiting room for outpatients and inpatients.

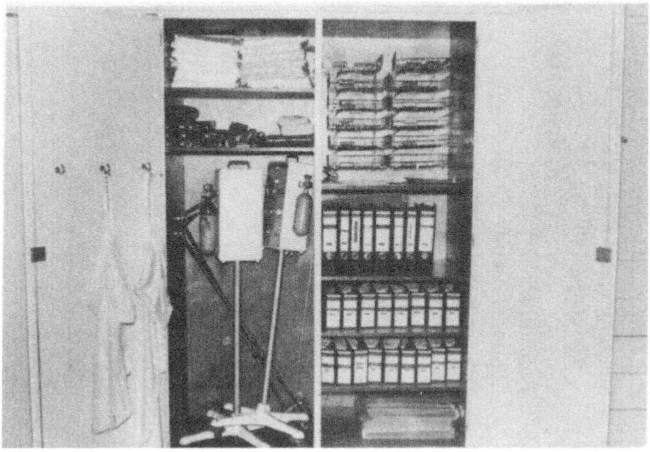

Fig. 6. Storage facility for written reports and X-ray films.

storage of instruments and reports, a desk and chair, and at least five electric outlets distributed throughout the room.

In hospitals and hospital departments where the number of endoscopic procedures exceeds 30 per week and where, in addition, specialized endoscopic procedures are carried out, several rooms should be available (Table 2). If different endoscopic procedures are performed in one room, consideration must be given to the requirements of asepsis, as well as to

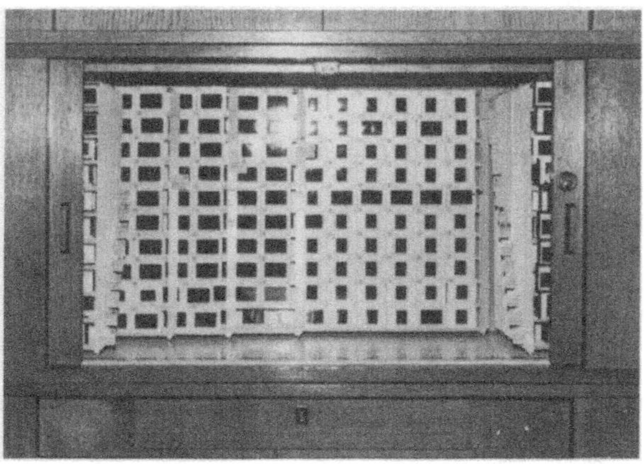

Fig. 7. Cabinet for viewing of slides with lateral compartments for storage of slides and movies (Bonacker, Bremen).

Table 2. Assignment of endoscopic procedures to one or several rooms.

Planning of endoscopy rooms

1 Room	2 Rooms		3 Rooms		
Laparoscopy	Laparoscopy	Esophagogastro-duodenoscopy	Laparoscopy	Esophagogastro-duodenoscopy	ERCP, EPT
Esophagogastro-duodenoscopy		Proctoscopy		Postbulbar duodenoscopy	Colonoscopy
Proctoscopy		Sigmoidoscopy		Proctoscopy	Ileoscopy
Sigmoidoscopy				Sigmoidoscopy	

4 Rooms			
Laparoscopy	Esophagogastro-duodenoscopy	ERCP, EPT	Proctoscopy
	Postbulbar duodenoscopy	Enteroscopy	Sigmoidoscopy
			Colonoscopy
			Ileoscopy

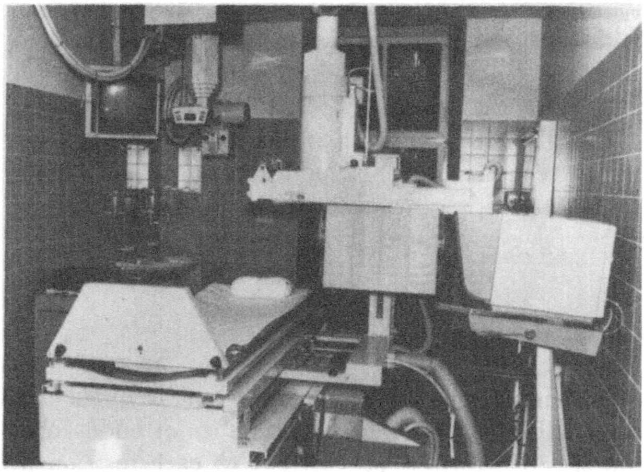

Fig. 8. X-ray unit (Sireskop 3 with Explorator 35, Siemens) with floating table top and image-intensifier TV monitor.

the frequency of examinations. Particular problems arise with those endoscopic procedures for which X-ray equipment is necessary [retrograde cholangiopancreatography (ERCP), papillotomy (EPT), angiography, enteroscopy] or desirable (colonoscopy).

Endoscopic procedures for which fluoroscopy or roentgenographic documentation is required can be performed in the X-ray department. Nevertheless, when the volume of examinations becomes large, the endoscopist needs access to an X-ray unit that is constantly available. This unit needs to be located within the endoscopy suite.

An X-ray unit particularly suited for combined endoscopic/radiologic examinations is a fluoroscopy unit with spot film device (Sireskop 3 and Explorator 35, Siemens) featuring an image intensifier and TV monitor (Fig. 8). A floating table top and a 70 × 70 mm camera attached to the image intensifier allow rapid adjustment of position and avoidance of time-consuming cassette exchange, both allowing uninterrupted radiographic documentation, particularly during dynamic phases of the examination. A standard (up to 35 × 35 cm) cassette changer, however, has to be available also, particularly for laparoscopic splenoportography and transhepatic cholangiography.

The effect of X-rays on fiberoptic endoscopes is of particular importance. Experiments performed under contract with Wappler International GmbH, Munich, have shown that a conventional fiberoptic endoscope can be used for about 800 h (exposure of 0.5 R/h) if one assumes 50% absorption of the radiation energy by the glass fiber bundle. An additional radiation shield in the area of the sleeve of some types of endoscopes may further reduce or eliminate this source of damage to the fiber bundles.

During construction or remodeling of an endoscopy section [3], one must decide whether to arrange the examining units in an open or closed fashion. The partial separation of the examining tables by curtains or freely mobile partitions appears less desirable because of the lack of noise insulation. A plan for the spatial arrangement and distribution of the functions of a modern endoscopy section, which also performs outpatient examinations, is shown in Fig. 9. This represents optimal conditions that can be modified depending on the space and money available.

1.1.2 Equipment and Instuments

As in the planning of the endoscopy rooms, the type and frequency of the endoscopic procedures will also determine the number of endoscopic instruments to be purchased. In principle, at least two of each instrument type should be available so that endoscopic procedures can be continued if one instrument fails. Table 3 lists the instruments required for office practice, community hospitals, and large medical centers with a gastroenterology department; the associated costs are shown in Tables 4–6. In each case these are optimal requirements. As minimal investment costs, one can assume about one-half of the listed prices (as of 1980); this will, however, provide an endoscopy unit with only limited functional capacity.

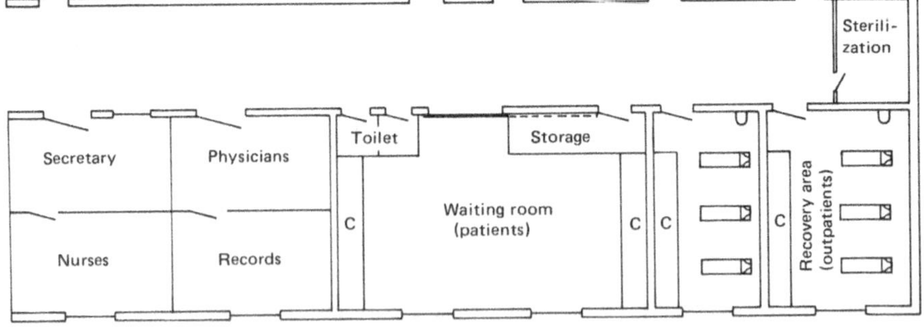

Fig. 9. Floor plan of a modern endoscopy section. Endoscopy room *I*, proctoscopy, colonoscopy, ileoscopy, sigmoidoscopy; *II*, ERCP, EPT, enteroscopy; *III*, esophagogastroduodenoscopy, postbulbar duodenoscopy; *IV*, laparoscopy. *C*, cabinet.

Table 3. Recommended equipment for endoscopy units in office practice, hospitals, and medical centers.

General practitioner/ internist	*Hospital*	*Medical (gastroenterology) center*
2 anoscopes	3 anoscopes	4 anoscopes
2 proctosigmoidoscopes	3 proctosigmoidoscopes	6 proctosigmoidoscopes
	3 liver biopsy trays (blind biopsy)	6 liver biopsy trays (blind biopsy)
	2 laparoscopes	4 laparoscopes
	2 small bowel biopsy capsules + 1 vacuum pump	3 small bowel biopsy capsules + 2 vacuum pumps
	2 esophagogastroduodeno-scopes	3 esophagogastroduodeno-scopes
	1 duodenoscope (side viewing)	3 duodenoscopes (side viewing)
	1 fibersigmoidoscope	1 sigmoidoscope
	1 colonoscope	3 colonoscopes
		Accessories for therapeutic endoscopy
		Teaching model
		Slide series (audiovisual training

Table 4. Equipment for endoscopy units in an office practice (as of 1980).

Equipment for: *Office practice (general practitioner, internist, surgeon)*	
2 anoscopes with accessories	600. DM[a]
2 proctosigmoidoscopes with accessories	1340. DM
1 light source and cable	1300. DM
Total	3240. DM

[a] Editor's note: The prices quoted in Tables 4–7 are based on current list prices (subject to change) in the Federal Republic of Germany. Since list prices vary in different countries, the DM (Deutsche Mark) amounts provide an approximate basis for calculating the necessary expenditure for the various equipment items.

Table 5. Instrument costs for endoscopy unit in a hospital (as of 1980).

Equipment with instruments: hospital	
3 anoscopes with accessories	750. DM
3 protosigmoidoscopes with accessories	1540. DM
1 light source with cable	1300. DM
3 liver biopsy trays with accessories (blind biopsy)	500. DM
2 laparoscopes with accessories	10 000. DM
2 small bowel biopsy capsules + 1 vacuum pump	2850. DM
2 esophagogastroduodenoscopes	37 100. DM
1 duodenoscope (side viewing)	18 800. DM
1 fibersigmoidoscope	17 000. DM
1 colonoscope	19 500. DM
1 light source	4000. DM
Accessories (forceps, cameras)	1500. DM
1 teaching attachment	5400. DM
Subtotal	120 240. DM
Emergency supplies for complications	400. DM
Equipment for manual ventilation	2000. DM
High frequency electrosurgery unit	3000. DM
CO_2 insufflator (Siede)	2270. DM
Total	127 910. DM

Although the price for the optimal equipment of an endoscopy section may appear to be high on first sight, the investment is actually small in comparison to other instruments used for diagnostic studies (X ray, nuclear medicine, clinical laboratory) as well as in relation to the diagnostic and therapeutic capabilities of the endoscopic methods. On the other hand, it should be stated that the fee of 25 DM for esophagogastroscopy, duodenojejunoscopy, colonoscopy, or laparoscopy listed in the official fee scale for physicians in Germany is inappropriate in relation to the actual costs (acquisition, depreciation, and repairs) (Table 7).

1.1.3 Staffing

The effectiveness and quality of an endoscopy section are determined by the expertise of the endoscopist and ancillary personnel in addition to the quality of the instruments. In view of the diversity of endoscopic biopsy findings and the technical difficulties of endoscopic procedures, only individuals with the necessary basic knowledge of the endoscopic techniques should perform these examinations. Familiarity with potential complications, their prevention, and the necessary countermeasures (page 35)

Table 6. Instrument costs for endoscopy unit in a medical center (as of 1980).

Equipment with instruments:		
Medical (gastroenterology) center		
Basic equipment (as in hospital)		127 910. DM
In addition		
1 anoscope without accessories		160. DM
3 proctosigmoidoscopes without accessories		600. DM
3 liver biopsy trays without accessories (blind biopsy)		470. DM
2 laparascopes without accessories		6480. DM
1 small bowel biopsy capsule without accessories		600. DM
1 esophagogastroduodenoscope		18 550. DM
2 duodenoscopes (side viewing)		37 600. DM
2 colonoscopes		39 000. DM
Accessories for therapeutic endoscopy (snares, forceps, etc.)		4000. DM
Teaching model		1500. DM
Slide series (audiovisual training)		500. DM
Subtotal	237 370. DM	
Expanded equipment		
Movie camera (16 mm)		4500. DM
Color television unit	45 000	— 150 000. DM
Movie light source		13 600. DM
Small X-ray unit (C loop with 70 mm camera)	168 000. DM	
X-ray unit (angiography, ductography, splenoportography and colonoscopy)		600 000. DM
Total	450 370. DM—	1 005 470. DM

is just as necessary as a basic knowledge of the lesions that one is likely to encounter [1,2]. The number of physicians performing endoscopy and of ancillary personnel will depend upon the number of examinations as well as the number of rooms in which the procedures can be performed simultaneously. If only one room is available, two physicians and two nurses who can replace each other should suffice. If, however, procedures are performed simultaneously, an endoscopist, a nurse, and an aide should

Table 7. Equipment costs for specific endoscopic examinations (Department of Medicine, University of Erlangen, 1978).

Esophagogastroduodenoscopy	213. DM
Duodenoscopy with retrograde cannulation	301. DM
Colonoscopy	188. DM
Laparoscopy	75. DM

be available for each room. A second physician needs to be present for those procedures that require fluoroscopic control or X-ray documentation (retrograde pancreatocholangiography, papillotomy, enteroscopy, angiography, splenoportography, and colonoscopy) and, occasionally, during laparoscopy. An emergency endoscopy service available 24 h a day requires at least four endoscopists and four nurses working weekly shifts.

References

1. Classen, M., Frühmorgen, P., Rösch, W.: Gastrointestinale Endoskopie: Versuch einer Bewertung. Internist (Berlin) *14*, 245 (1973)
2. Morson, B. C.: Histological typing of intestinal tumours: World Health Organization, Geneva, 1976
3. Ottenjann, R.: Die gastroenterologische Abteilung im Stadt- und Kreiskrankenhaus. Fortschr. Med. *91*, 866 (1973)

1.2

Cleaning and Maintenance of Endoscopic Instruments

R. HOHNER/CHR. ROMFELD

Hygiene in an endoscopy section is mainly directed at disinfection, sterilization, and control of nosocomial infections [2,5,6]. The cleaning of our instruments is based on the principles of disinfection (Table 1) and sterilization (Table 2) [3]. All fiberendoscopic instruments first undergo preliminary disinfection and are then cleaned, disinfected, or sterilized (Table 3). Three types of instruments must be distinguished:

Table 1. Disinfection in endoscopy.

Chemically (20–30 min) by	*Physically* (20–30 min) by	
Tested disinfecting agents:	Heat:	UV rays:
For fiberendoscopes, heat-sensitive instruments, apparatus, and endoscopy rooms	For heat-resistant instruments	Room disinfection

Table 2. Sterilization in endoscopy.

Physically by		*Chemically* by
Heat		Ethylene oxide gas (alternative: glutaraldehyde)
Hot air 180° C:	Pressurized steam (autoclave 134° C):	For optics, heat-sensitive materials
For syringes, needles, glassware	For surgical instruments, linen, optics, syringes, needles	

Table 3. Procedure for endoscopic instruments.

Predisinfection 10–20 min
Gigasept 5%* and M & S Labor** 2%

Cleaning and rinsing
M & S Labor**, distilled water

Disinfection
Gigasept 10%* (10 min–4½ h)
Alhydex (10 min–3 h)
(gluteraldehyde)

Rinsing in distilled water
Drying (pressurized air up to 0.5 atm)

Sterilization
Pressurized steam 134° C
Hot air 180° C

Ethylene oxide gas

Storage and venting

Other commercially available disinfecting agents have not yet been evaluated by us.

* Gigasept: Succindialdehyde, dimethoxytetrahydrofuran, formaldehyde
** M&S Labor: Tenside, phosphate, carbonate

1.2.1 Instruments That Can Be Sterilized by Various Procedures Without Restrictions

Surgical instruments, biopsy needles, trocars, syringes and containers, glassware, and tubing material that can be autoclaved are placed immediately after use into a self-cleansing 5% disinfectant solution for 10 min and are cleaned manually afterward. Modern clinics provide automatic instrument washers. Needles for pneumoperitoneum and biopsies must be checked for patency and for damage of the tip prior to sterilization. The instruments are assembled on ready-to-use trays for the individual examinations (Fig. 1, Deponetten-System/Martin). Sterilization of the instruments can be accomplished by hot air or pressurized steam (Table 2).

1.2.2 Instruments with Limited Tolerance for Sterilization

Due to their construction or the nature of the materials utilized, only certain methods of disinfection and sterilization can be employed for rigid endoscopes, fiberoptic light cables, polypectomy loops, biopsy forceps, catheters, and papillotomes.

Cleaning and disinfection of rigid endoscopes does not create any problems (Table 1). The construction of laparoscopes, bronchoscopes, esophagoscopes, and proctoscopes is easy to understand; hence, they can be easily dismantled. After use, all parts are placed in a self-cleansing disinfectant solution, and the biopsy channels of the rigid endoscopes are

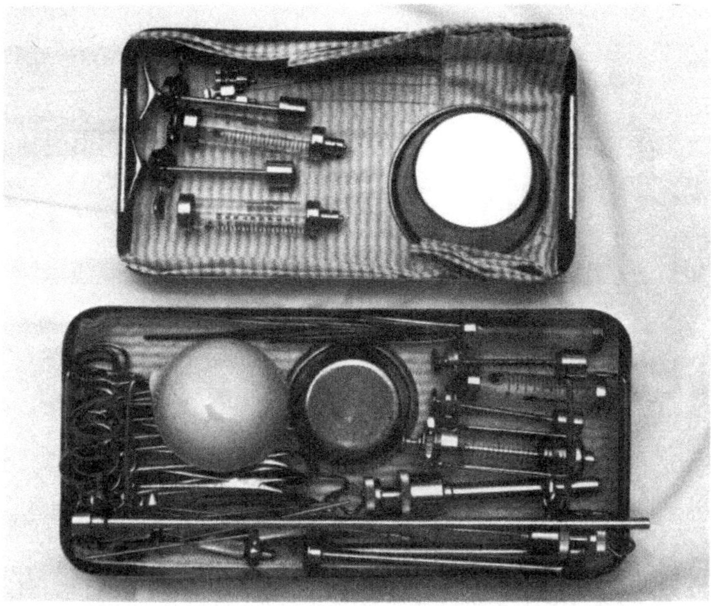

Fig. 1. Instruments that can be sterilized without restrictions.

cleaned with a brush and cleaning pistol (Selecta). It is important to remove adherent residues of blood and serum, oil and fat particles, as well as inorganic substances. After disinfection and cleaning have been accomplished, the instruments are rinsed with distilled water. Prior to sterilization one must pay particular attention to the objective and ocular surfaces and to the light entry and exit surfaces of the light channels and fiber cables. Residual contamination can be removed by rubbing with soap and moist cotton balls. Rubber caps and baskets can fulfill their assigned role only if their holes have the correct size and show no tears. Hinges of stopcocks must be greased with special oil. After the instruments have been examined for possible damage, they are double-wrapped in towels, test tapes with dates are attached, and the instruments are gas- or steam-sterilized in the appropriate containers according to the manufacturer's recommendations. An alternative is chemical sterilization. The exposure time is 3–4½ h. Proctoscopes are treated separately from all other instruments to avoid the spread of pathogens.

The manual cleaning of biopsy forceps and polypectomy snares, rather small instruments of complicated shape, requires a considerable amount of time every day, and small nooks and crannies cannot be reached adequately. A better cleaning effect can be accomplished by ultrasound. Ultrasound vibrations generate tiny bubbles in the cleaning solution which

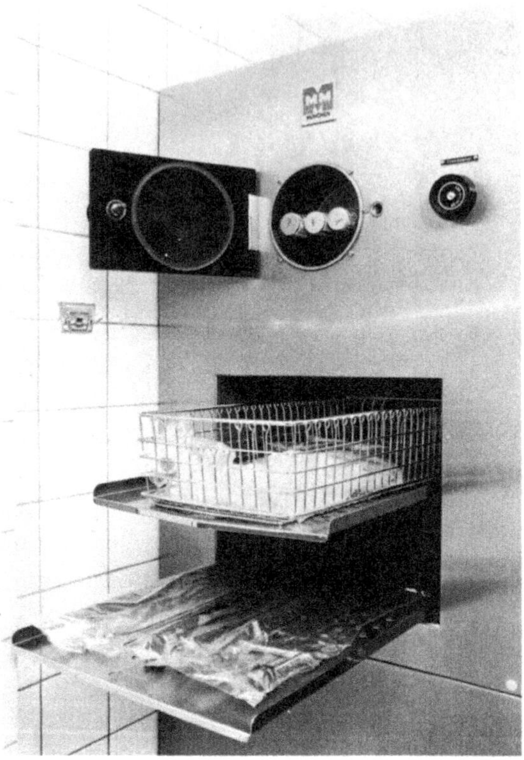

Fig. 2. Gas-sterilization of instruments that can be sterilized with restrictions only.

exert mechanical cleaning forces during implosion. Ultrasound cleaning devices have been designed particularly for the removal of contamination invisible to the human eye. Crusts tend to form on the surface during use of coagulation electrodes, polypectomy snares, and papillotomes. This layer can be removed by scrubbing with fine sandpaper. These temperature-sensitive products, as well as special catheters and probes, should be sealed after drying in transparent foils of 0.03-mm thickness and subsequently gas-sterilized (Fig. 2).

1.2.3 Instruments That Can Be Sterilized Only Under Exceptional Circumstances

Flexible fiber endoscopes cannot be disinfected adequately and sterilized after each examination (Table 3). In contrast to the instruments already mentioned, they cannot be dismantled. The air and biopsy channels are poorly accessible for cleaning. Moreover, the instrument control handle should not be exposed to water. After use of a fiberoptic endoscope, the rubber caps are removed and adherent mucus and blood are wiped off; the instrument is then carefully washed under running water; the biopsy channel is brushed and flushed. This preliminary disinfection is carried out in a 5% disinfectant solution (Gigasept) with a 2% cleaning agent as an additive (M&S Labor). Thereafter, the fiberoptic endoscopes are disinfected. During this process, the instrument channels as well as the outside of the endoscope should be carefully rinsed with the disinfectant solution; it is best to fill the biopsy and air channels with the disinfecting agent and to submerge the instrument, except for the handle and the connecting cable, in the solution for 15–20 min (Fig. 3). No air bubbles should remain in the channels since they interfere with the process of disinfection. Protein remnants also have adverse effects by inactivating the disinfecting solution. Afterward, the endoscopes are flushed with distilled water. Contrary to the

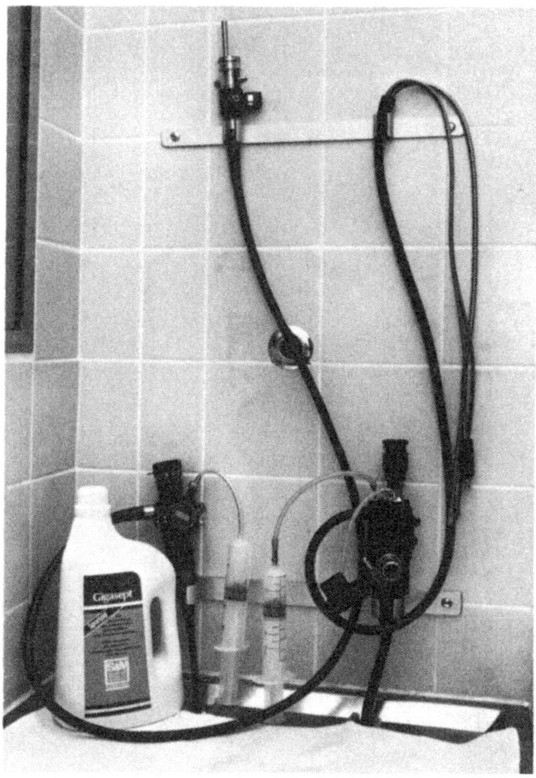

Fig. 3. Disinfection of fiber endoscopes.

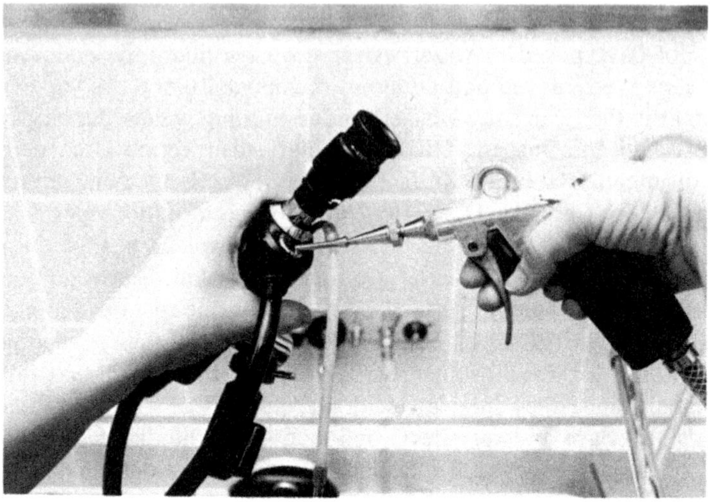

Fig. 4. Flushing of endoscope channels with distilled water.

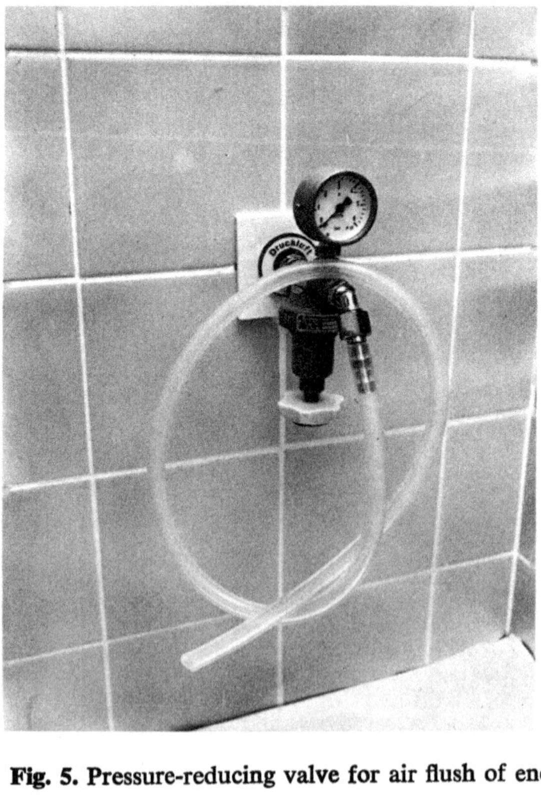

Fig. 5. Pressure-reducing valve for air flush of endoscopy channels.

recommendations of the manufacturers, we use a Selecta spray gun with a particularly fine nozzle for this purpose. We hold it against the openings of the suction and air buttons or channels and flush under low pressure (Fig. 4). Fully automated disinfecting instruments for fiberoptic endoscopes have recently been developed. The working principle of these instruments consists of a recirculating flush arrangement of all channels of the fiberoptic endoscope. The turnover time of the disinfecting agent can be selected in steps of 1, 5, 10, 15, 20, and 30 min [4].

After these disinfection steps, the fiberoptic endoscopes are carefully dried and all residual humidity removed from the connecting tubes and biopsy channels. If pressurized air is used, we do not exceed 0.5 atm (Fig. 5, pressure reducing valve/Draeger). In addition, corrosions in the plug adapter of the service channel are removed and gaskets renewed.

A check of all functions of the instrument is part of a careful preparation for endoscopy. Regular, careful inspection of the endoscopes and correction of small defects help to prevent larger repairs. An example is a small triangular tear in the rubber cuff of the instrument tip caused by a tooth. Replacement of the rubber cuff is a small repair; water entry may become expensive. The fiber endoscopes are stored either lying in appropriate drawers or hanging in cabinets (Fig. 6). Colonoscopes with accessories are treated and stored separately from all other instruments.

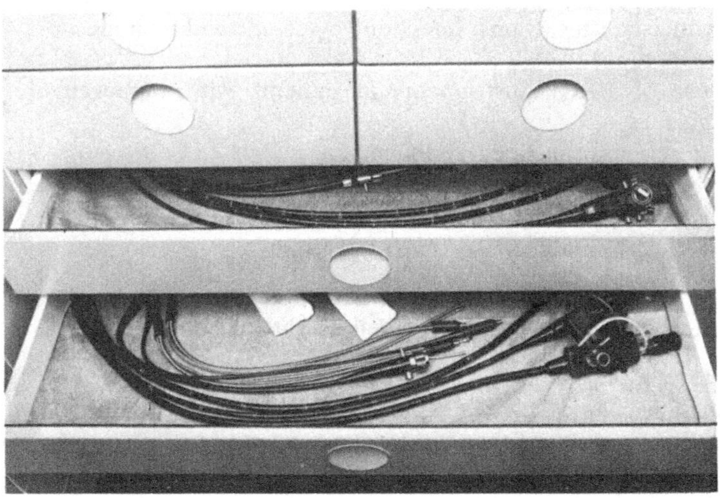

Fig. 6. Storage of fiber endoscopes.

1.2.4 Nosocomial Infections

Endoscopy sections should be considered as diagnostic units with a high potential for infectivity [1]. Even thorough manual cleaning and disinfection of the fiber endoscopes can only reach a degree of cleanliness that satisfies aesthetic demands. This is due to their complicated structure, in particular due to the long channels equipped with valves. Based on bacteriologic studies, the transmission of organisms during several successive endoscopic examinations is at least theoretically possible. The physician, therefore, should decide whether he wants to disinfect the fiber endoscopes completely at least once a day, which would require several hours to achieve a relative level of safety, eliminating highly resistant bacteria and viruses.

Sterilization cannot be accomplished routinely at the present time because of the nature of the structural materials. Although our studies indicate that fiberoptic endoscopes can be sterilized with ethylene oxide [7], the procedure is rather cumbersome. Moreover, the endoscope is out of use for about 24–48 h, which are required for sterilization and ventilation. Gas-sterilization is, however, mandatory under the following conditions:

1) After contamination of the endoscope with infectious material (*Salmonella*, tubercle bacilli, hepatitis viruses, *Spirochaeta pallida*)
2) For endoscopy of particularly susceptible patients with impaired defense mechanisms against infection (cytostatic and immunosuppressive therapy)
3) After use of ERCP instruments in patients with suppurative cholangitis
4) For endoscopy in an open abdomen
5) Once a week, for instance, on weekends, if the instrument is used daily, as a compromise between the demands of the epidemiologist and practical limitations

Maximum cleanliness must prevail in an endoscopy section to prevent nosocomial infections. The following guidelines should be observed:

a) Separate handling of septic and aseptic instruments
b) Thorough mechanical cleaning and disinfection
c) Sterilization of material that can be sterilized easily
d) Gas-sterilization of fiberoptic instruments in selected cases

References

1. Bass, E. U.: Fiberendoskop-Desinfektion—ein ungelöstes Problem? Aktuel. Gastrol. *6*(4), 307–314 (1977)

2. Deming, L.: Significance and current status of disinfection in gastroenterological endoscopy. Endoscopy *10*, 69–70 (1978)
3. Kanz, E.: Aseptik in der Chirurgie. Stuttgart: Thieme 1973
4. Nemethy, G.: Instrumentation: Cleaning, storage, and maintenance and supervision of endoscopes. In: Endoscopy. Berci, G. (ed.), p. 133–154. New York: Appleton-Century-Crofts 1976
5. Slotnick, I. J.: Microbiology and sterilization of endoscopes. In: Endoscopy. Berci, G. (ed.) p. 155–172. New York: Appleton-Century-Crofts 1976
6. Tolon, M., Thofern, E., Miederer, S. E.: Disinfection procedures of fiberscopes in endoscopy departments. Endoscopy *8*, 24–19 (1976)
7. Ujeyl, A. K., Wurbs, D., Adam, W., Classen, M.: Gassterilization of Fiber Endoscopes. Endoscopy *10*, 71–74 (1978)

1.3
Documentation of Endoscopic Findings

P. FRÜHMORGEN

Endoscopic findings can be documented in writing (longhand, punch card, computer) as well as in visual form (drawing, 35-mm camera, Polaroid camera, Super 8 and 16-mm movies, X ray) [1,8]. Visual documentation alone, however, is only an incomplete substitute for a written report [7].

1.3.1 Written Report

All endoscopic findings must be documented immediately upon completion of the examination. This can be done either directly in the patient record or by a separate report dictated on tape. The purpose of the written report is interpretation of the findings and their overall assessment. As a rule, one should avoid time-consuming descriptions of details that can be documented better by objective visual means [1].

1.3.2 Punch Cards

For statistical evaluation, a marginal punch card has proved to be useful (Figs. 1–3). All information of possible interest for future evaluation, listed in the margins of the card, is checked off immediately after the examination and is punched later. Additional information can be written in longhand on the center of the card (front and back side). Sketches or rubber stamps have proved to be useful to indicate the location of findings (Figs. 4 and 5).

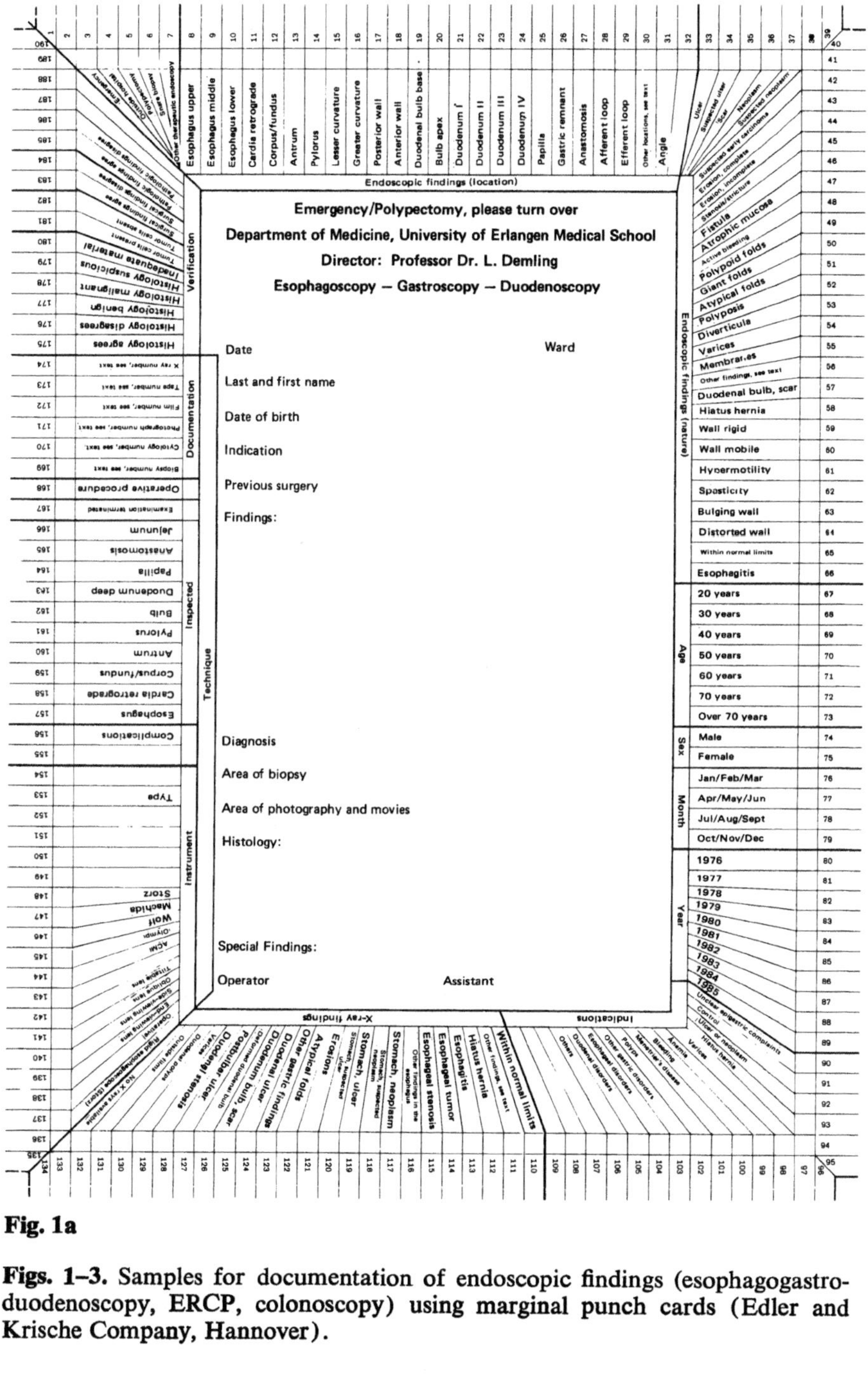

Fig. 1a

Figs. 1–3. Samples for documentation of endoscopic findings (esophagogastroduodenoscopy, ERCP, colonoscopy) using marginal punch cards (Edler and Krische Company, Hannover).

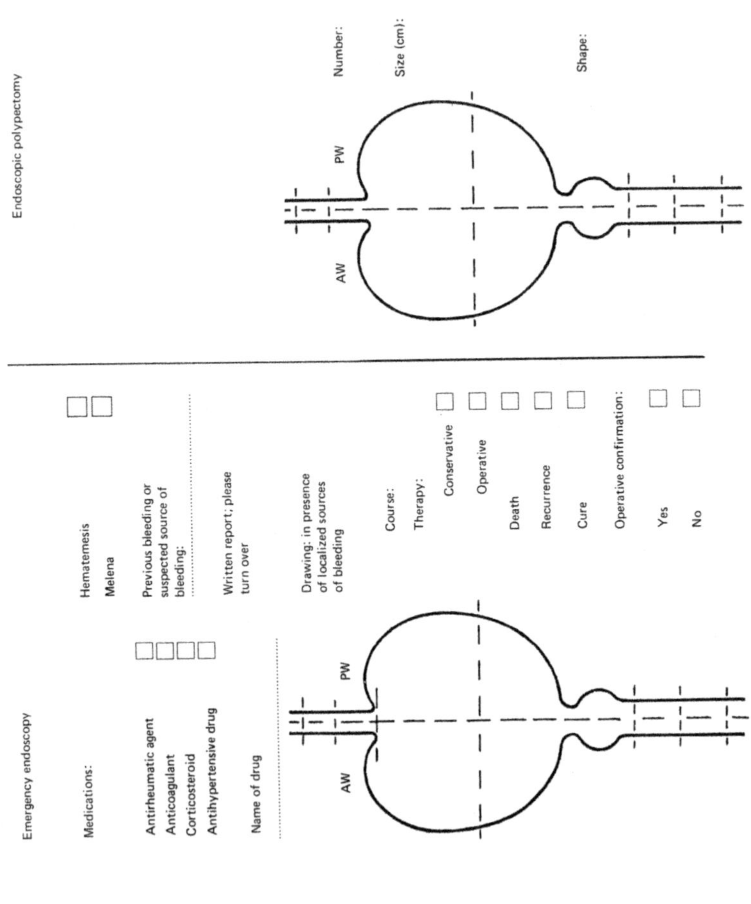

Fig. 1b. Back side of Fig. 1a.

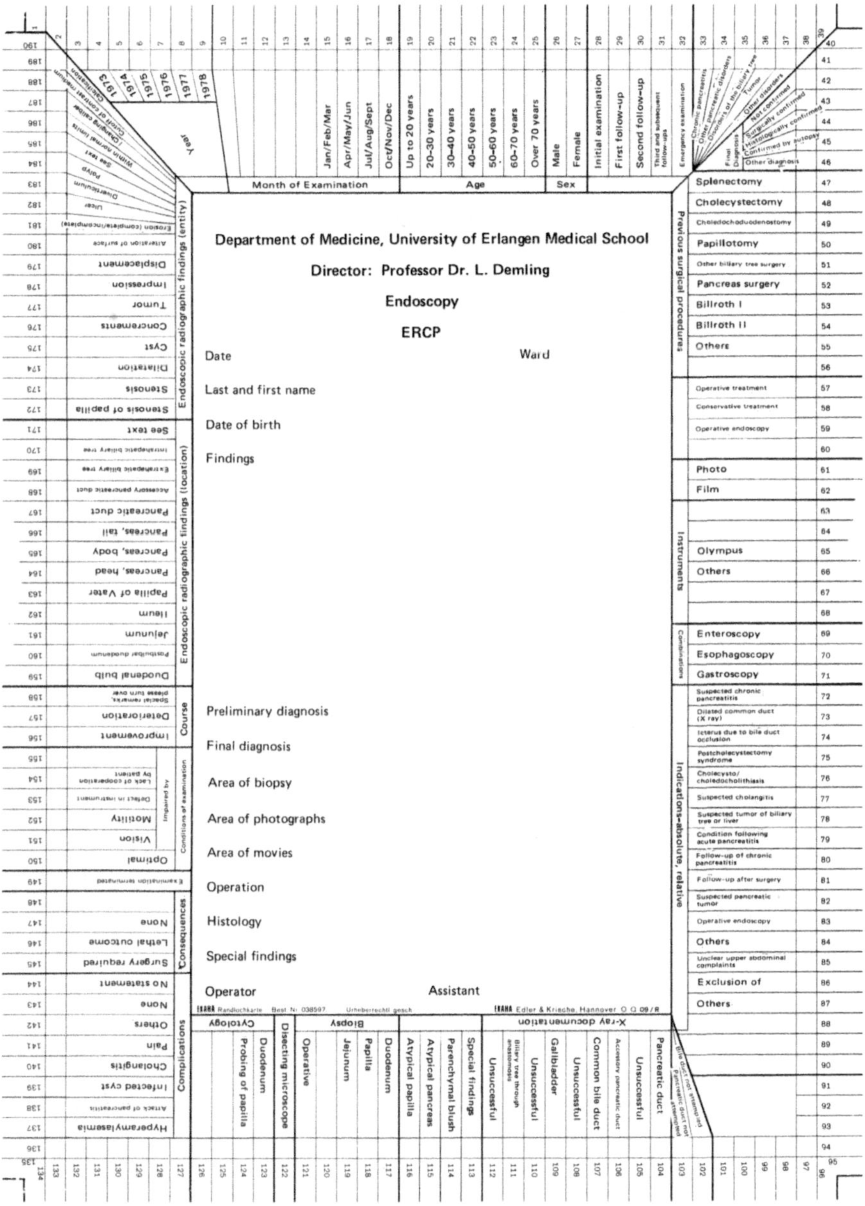
Department of Medicine, University of Erlangen Medical School

Director: Professor Dr. L. Demling

Endoscopy

ERCP

Date Ward

Last and first name

Date of birth

Findings

Preliminary diagnosis

Final diagnosis

Area of biopsy

Area of photographs

Area of movies

Operation

Histology

Special findings

Operator Assistant

Year: 1973, 1974, 1975, 1976, 1977, 1978

Month of Examination: Jan/Feb/Mar, Apr/May/Jun, Jul/Aug/Sept, Oct/Nov/Dec

Age: Up to 20 years, 20–30 years, 30–40 years, 40–50 years, 50–60 years, 60–70 years, Over 70 years

Sex: Male, Female

Initial examination, First follow-up, Second follow-up, Third and subsequent follow-ups, Emergency examination

Final Diagnosis: Chronic pancreatitis, Other pancreatic disorders, Disorders of the biliary tree, Tumor, Other disorders, Not confirmed, Surgically confirmed, Histologically confirmed, Confirmed by autopsy, Other diagnosis

Previous surgical procedures: Splenectomy, Cholecystectomy, Choledochoduodenostomy, Papillotomy, Other biliary tree surgery, Pancreas surgery, Billroth I, Billroth II, Others

Operative treatment, Conservative treatment, Operative endoscopy

Photo, Film

Instruments: Olympus, Others

Combinations: Enteroscopy, Esophagoscopy, Gastroscopy

Indications-absolute, relative: Suspected chronic pancreatitis, Dilated common duct (X ray), Icterus due to bile duct occlusion, Postcholecystectomy syndrome, Cholecysto/choledocholithiasis, Suspected cholangitis, Suspected tumor of biliary tree or liver, Condition following acute pancreatitis, Follow-up of chronic pancreatitis, Follow-up after surgery, Suspected pancreatic tumor, Operative endoscopy, Others, Unclear upper abdominal complaints, Exclusion of, Others

X-ray documentation: Pancreatic duct, Unsuccessful, Accessory pancreatic duct, Common bile duct, Unsuccessful, Gallbladder, Unsuccessful, Biliary tree through anastomosis, Unsuccessful, Bile duct not attempted, Pancreatic duct not attempted

Special findings, Parenchymal blush, Atypical pancreas, Atypical papilla

Biopsy: Duodenum, Papilla, Jejunum, Operative

Dissecting microscope

Cytology: Duodenum, Probing of papilla

Complications: Hyperamylasemia, Attack of pancreatitis, Infected cyst, Cholangitis, Pain, Others, None, No statement

Consequences: Surgery required, Lethal outcome, None

Examination terminated

Conditions of examination: Optimal, Vision, Motility, Impaired by: Defect in instrument, Lack of cooperation by patient

Course: Improvement, Deterioration, Special remarks, please turn over

Endoscopic radiographic findings (location): Duodenal bulb, Postbulbar duodenum, Jejunum, Ileum, Papilla of Vater, Pancreas, head, Pancreas, body, Pancreas, tail, Pancreatic duct, Accessory pancreatic duct, Extrahepatic biliary tree, Intrahepatic biliary tree, See text

Endoscopic radiographic findings (entity): Stenosis of papilla, Stenosis, Dilatation, Cyst, Concrements, Tumor, Impression, Displacement, Alteration of surface, Erosion (complete/incomplete), Ulcer, Diverticulum, Polyp, See text, Within normal limits, Changing caliber, Cutoff of contrast medium, Calcification

Randlochkarte Best. Nr. 038597 Urheberrecht gesch. Edler & Krische, Hannover

Fig. 2

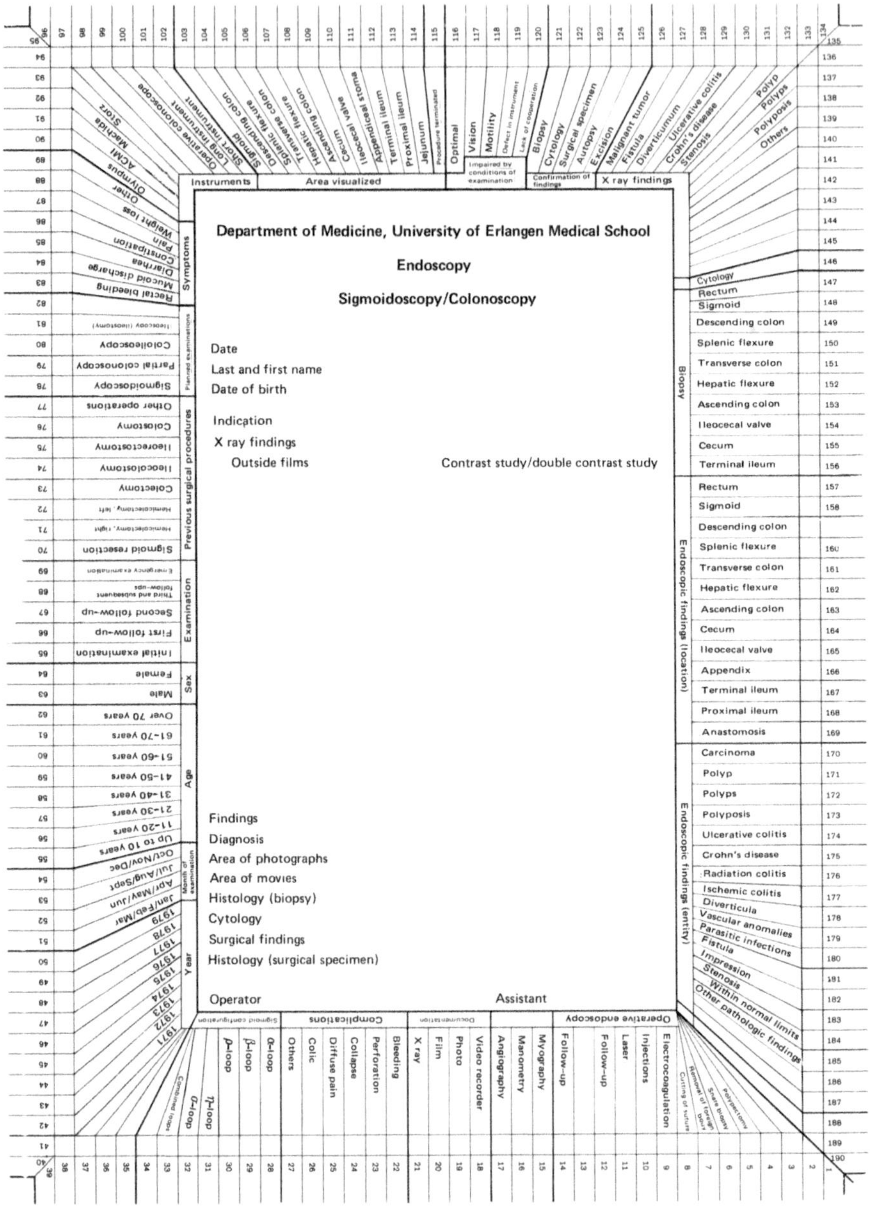

Department of Medicine, University of Erlangen Medical School
Endoscopy
Sigmoidoscopy/Colonoscopy
Date
Last and first name
Date of birth
Indication
X ray findings
Outside films
Contrast study/double contrast study
Findings
Diagnosis
Area of photographs
Area of movies
Histology (biopsy)
Cytology
Surgical findings
Histology (surgical specimen)
Operator
Assistant
Instruments
Storz
Machida
ACMI
Olympus
Other
Operative colonoscope
Long instrument
Short instrument
Area visualized
Sigmoid colon
Descending colon
Splenic flexure
Transverse colon
Hepatic flexure
Ascending colon
Cecum
Ileocecal valve
Appendiceal stoma
Terminal ileum
Proximal ileum
Jejunum
Procedure terminated
Optimal
Vision
Motility
Defect in instrument
Lack of cooperation
Impaired by conditions of examination
Biopsy
Cytology
Surgical specimen
Autopsy
Excision
Confirmation of findings
Malignant tumor
Fistula
Diverticulum
Crohn's disease
Ulcerative colitis
Stenosis
Polyp
Polyps
Polyposis
Others
X ray findings
Symptoms
Weight loss
Pain
Constipation
Diarrhea
Mucoid discharge
Rectal bleeding
Planned examinations
Ileoscopy (ileostomy)
Colileoscopy
Partial colonoscopy
Sigmoidoscopy
Previous surgical procedures
Other operations
Colostomy
Ileorectostomy
Ileocolostomy
Colectomy
Hemicolectomy, left
Hemicolectomy, right
Sigmoid resection
Examination
Emergency examination
Third and subsequent follow-ups
Second follow-up
First follow-up
Initial examination
Sex
Female
Male
Age
Over 70 years
61-70 years
51-60 years
41-50 years
31-40 years
21-30 years
11-20 years
Up to 10 years
Month of examination
Oct/Nov/Dec
Jul/Aug/Sept
Apr/May/Jun
Jan/Feb/Mar
Year
1979
1978
1977
1976
1975
1974
1973
1972
1971
Biopsy
Cytology
Rectum
Sigmoid
Descending colon
Splenic flexure
Transverse colon
Hepatic flexure
Ascending colon
Ileocecal valve
Cecum
Terminal ileum
Endoscopic findings (location)
Rectum
Sigmoid
Descending colon
Splenic flexure
Transverse colon
Hepatic flexure
Ascending colon
Cecum
Ileocecal valve
Appendix
Terminal ileum
Proximal ileum
Anastomosis
Endoscopic findings (entity)
Carcinoma
Polyp
Polyps
Polyposis
Ulcerative colitis
Crohn's disease
Radiation colitis
Ischemic colitis
Diverticula
Vascular anomalies
Parasitic infections
Fistula
Impression
Stenosis
Within normal limits
Other pathologic findings
Sigmoid configuration
Combined loops
Ω-loop
η-loop
ρ-loop
β-loop
α-loop
Complications
Others
Colic
Diffuse pain
Collapse
Perforation
Bleeding
Documentation
X ray
Film
Photo
Video recorder
Angiography
Manometry
Myography
Follow-up
Follow-up
Operative endoscopy
Laser
Injections
Electrocoagulation
Cutting of suture
Removal of foreign body
Snare biopsy
Polypectomy

Fig. 3a

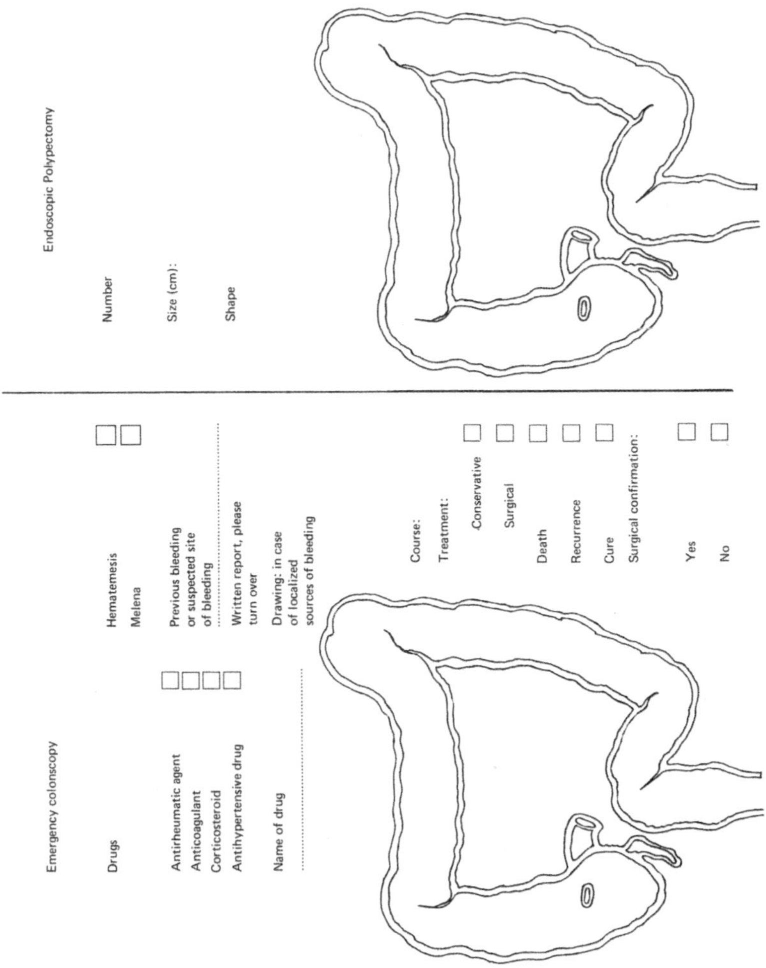

Fig. 3b. Back side of Fig. 3a.

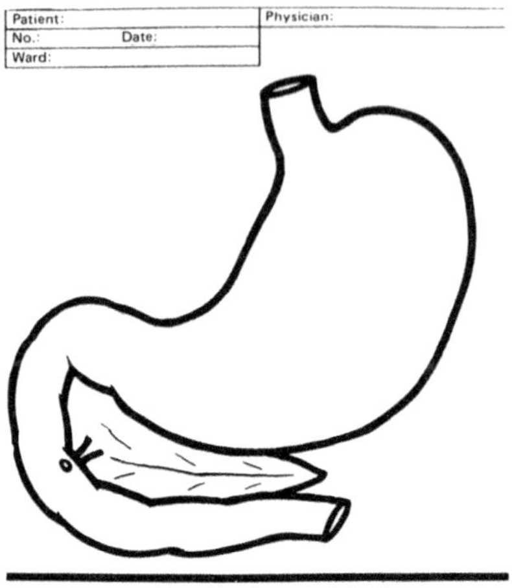

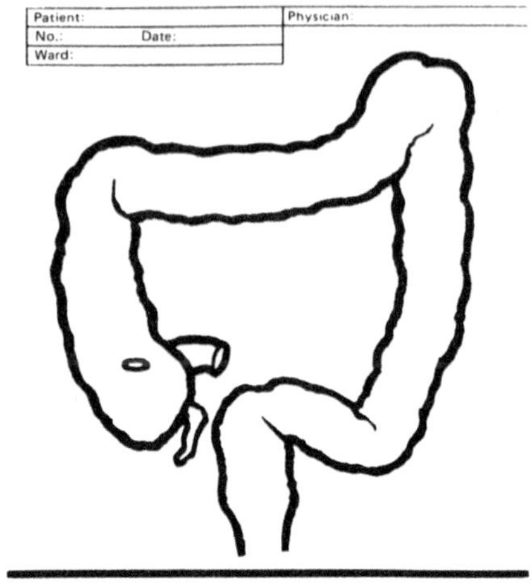

Figs. 4 and 5. Diagrams for the recording of pathologic findings.

1.3.3 Visual Documentation

Objective visual documentation can be accomplished by drawings, photography, movies, and, in special cases, radiography. The advances in color photography have made the drawing of pictures almost superfluous. Visual documention is used mainly for follow-up examinations, training and continuing education, as well as for therapeutic trials. This procedure has been particularly useful when different physicians examine the patient and also as a check on young endoscopists. In every case, however, photographic documentation should be combined with tissue biopsy for histologic confirmation of the diagnosis. Photo documentation alone is only of limited value as a diagnostic tool. For a description of the macroscopic findings, however, photography is superior to a written report, provided that the true colors are reproduced. Interpretation and definite statements about the clinical nature of the findings must be supported by histologic and cytologic studies.

While the quality of laparoscopic and sigmoidoscopic photography with rigid instruments had been satisfactory, color photographs through fiberoptic instruments did not reach the desired quality (brightness, power of resolution) for a long time. Intragastric photography (gastrocamera) is independent of some of these interfering factors (brightness, fiberoptics, adapter). For some time, therefore, it was considered the optimal form of gastrophotography. Due to the high quality of the fiberoptic systems, extragastric photography has now reached, and in some cases even surpassed, the quality of intragastric photographic systems. It, therefore, can now be used without loss of detailed information [2,3,5,6].

The intragastric camera without visual control can no longer be recommended for documentation of endoscopic findings because of the lower quality of the pictures (power of resolution, structural detail, distortion) and because it does not permit removal of tissue under direct vision for diagnostic purposes [2,3].

The described method of photo documentation has the distinct disadvantage that the photographs taken are not available for several days. Polaroid photographs developed within 1–2 min, however, cannot yet be recommended because of the sometimes inaccurate reproduction of color tones and the poor resolution of detail (small image).

The most common errors made during extragastric photography and their prevention include:

a) Incorrect setting of the exposure time.
b) Disregard for the depth of field (the given values are marginal values). The distance to be selected (i.e., the distance of the point of maximal focus from the anterior main plane of the objective) corresponds approximately to the middle between the indicated limits.
c) Insufficient lighting (in particular, in organs with a large lumen). By keeping air insufflation to a minimum, one should attempt to keep the organ cavity and the distance between object and lens at a minimum.
d) Insufficient cleaning of object, objective, and ocular. Checking the optical system prior to the examination as well as flushing during the procedure, preferably with dimethylpolysiloxane (Mylicon) in the presence of foam, can obviate these interfering factors.
e) Incorrect film material: daylight films for high-intensity cold light sources (Olympus CLX, CLS; ACMI 1010A) or flashlight; films for artificial light with weak light sources or hot light. The sensitivity indicated by the ASA number of the film determines the exposure time to be selected. Films with low ASA numbers, such as Agfachrome (professional) and Agfa CT 18 with 50 ASA, reproduce colors very well; the longer exposure times required for good illumination, however, will easily result in blurring due to motion. This can be avoided by using high-speed films (Kodak Ektachrome 160 ASA) and by having the patient hold his breath during photography.
f) If one suspects that the film was underexposed, one can adjust the sensitivity of the film by special processing ("ASA 100 proc-

essing," Agfa Gaevert Processing Laboratory, Inc., P.O. Box 711, Flushing, N.Y. 11352 or process E-4 adjustments for Ektachrome films). Brightening of already developed slides is also possible later on. This procedure, however, is expensive and therefore can be performed only for photographs of particular interest.

g) If instruments with adjustable focus are being used, focusing must be done manually after the object is in sight.

1.3.4 Technique of Photography with Extragastric Camera Using an Olympus Light Source

The light source runs constantly under full power. A light-absorbing grid is interposed during visual inspection; it is electronically controlled through the trigger and is removed from the light path during the exposure period, making the full light power available for photography. In the presence of a fixed exposure time in the camera (¼ s = 4), the actual exposure time required is computed through a photosensor and automatically adjusted (¼–1/100 s), depending on the distance between object and lens.

The camera with exchangeable or fixed adapter is firmly attached to the ocular of the endoscope by a twisting motion. A metal pin arrests the rotation and brings the ocular of the endoscope, adjusted to the eye of the examiner, into the zero position required for photography; in other words, the ocular of the endoscope is focused on the plane of the film by this manipulation. The optimal focus must be readjusted manually only in endoscopes with a variable focus, as mentioned above. Attention should be paid to the choice of the correct exposure time (¼ s) and to the tight fit of the synchronization cable.

The choice of the exposure index at the light source depends upon the film employed. The index can be used to alter the exposure time prior to shooting; adjustment to the film sensitivity is thereby possible (step 1 = longest exposure time, step 5 = shortest exposure time). Accordingly, steps 4 and 5 are suitable for high-speed films, steps 1 and 2 for less sensitive films. For Ektachrome 160 ASA film, one should select step 3; with a new CLE light source from Olympus (violet circle at the adjuster), step 4 should be dialed. The exposure time for the Agfa CT 18 film must be prolonged (steps 1 or 2) due to relatively low sensitivity.

If illumination of the object is unsatisfactory, the described electronic grid is not removed from the light path (absence of a click in the light source). Consequently, the film will be underexposed. To overcome this, one can shorten the distance between object and lens or dial a lower exposure index.

1.3.5 Technique of Automatic Photography with Extragastric Camera Using an ACMI Light Source

Needed for simplified automatic photography with an ACMI endoscope are a 35-mm camera (Contax RTS), a camera adapter, a flexible endoscope of the FX or TX series, and a powerful cold light source (1010A).

The camera is mounted on the ocular portion of the endoscope with an adapter that automatically focuses the ocular on the film plane. Kodak Ektachrome EH film with 160 ASA rating is recommended. The film speed on the camera must be set at 400 ASA. The same dial is used to correct for anticipated under- or overexposure. For automatic operation, one should dial position 1X and then set the exposure time (right upper corner of the camera) to the "automatic" position. A microcomputer in the camera will then measure and select the correct exposure time. Adjustment of distance and F stop are unnecessary. For photography, one only has to switch on the photolight at the cold light source.

Lenses with an appropriate adapter can also be used; however, this is morc cumbersome and prone to malfunction. During photography the ocular must be brought into "normal position" (the ocular will snap into position by turning). The lens must be set at infinity and the F stop opened as far as possible (with standard lenses, for instance, 2.8).

1.3.6 Slides of X-ray Films

It is possible to make slides from X-ray films. The simplest method is to use a single lens reflex camera, using a well-illuminated viewbox. Photography with a Leica camera through a Reprovit (tripod and ocular) made by Leitz is more cumbersome and expensive.

Film material: one can either go from a negative film (Agfa IFF 25 ASA) to a positive film or, preferably, use the Agfa-Dia-Direct film (32 ASA) which gives better contrast. An exposure meter should always be used.

1.3.7 Filing of Slides

The slide binding should be marked with serial number, year, name, and diagnosis (Fig. 6). The logging in a file according to diagnosis or name will facilitate the retrieval of the slides. Storage in a slide cabinet which features slide-carrying frames that can be placed in front of a built-in light screen, arranged by organ designations (A. Bonacker KG, Bremen-Lesum), is recommended.

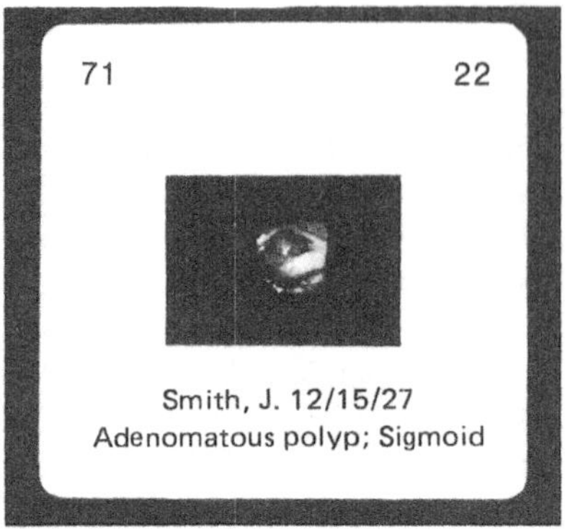

Fig. 6. Labeling of slides.

References

1. Beck, K., Dischler, W., Helms, M.: Die Bilddokumentation in der gastroenterologischen Endoskopie. Med. Welt *20*, 2573 (1969)
2. Frühmorgen, P., Demling, L., Seiler, C. F., Classen, M.: Gastrophotography–Gastroscopy. Endoscopy *4*, 133 (1972)
3. Frühmorgen, P., Habermalz, F., Demling, L., Haselmann, H.: The Efficiency of Gastrophotographic Systems. An experimental study. Endoscopy *5*, 1 (1973)
4. Haase, E.: Der Verwendungsbereich für Farbfilm in der Endoskopie. In: Demling, L., Ottenjann, R. (Ed.). Endoskopie, Methoden und Ergebnisse. Munich: Werk-Verlag 1969
5. Lindner, H.: Leistungsvermögen der Glasfaseroptiken. Z. Gastroenterol. *10*, 387 (1972)
6. Lindner, H., Fintelmann, V.: Systematik der Oesophago-, Gastro- und Bulboskope, Leber, Magen, Darm *1*, 155 (1971)
7. Oshima, H.: Gastrokamera-Untersuchung. Berlin: de Gruyter 1971
8. Winter, P., Heinkel, K.: Die Dokumentation endoskopischer Magenbefunde. In: Grundlagen der gastroenterologischen Endoskopie. Congress issue Nr. 1, Zeitschrift für Gastroenterologie. Heinkel, H. (Ed.). Gräfelfing: Demeter Verlag 1970

1.4
Emergency Treatment of Complications

W. RÖSCH

Even strict observation of absolute and relative contraindications does not always prevent complications during endoscopic procedures. Most accidents, however, can be traced to disregard for contraindications, among which lack of patient cooperation plays a particular role. In case of complications, the endoscopist should consider himself responsible for the further care of the patient. In case of an accident during an examination, repair and restoration of vital functions have absolute priority over completion of the examination, so that the patient will not be subjected to further risks unnecessarily.

Every endoscopist should be familiar with the possible complications of each procedure and he should be capable of initiating the necessary emergency treatment. It is essential to know where the necessary drugs are located and how to intubate and resuscitate an unconscious patient immediately.

1.4.1 Endoscopy of the Upper Digestive Tract

Reactions to topical anesthetics, generally applied prior to introduction of the instrument, are unpredictable and cannot be prevented by intracutaneous or conjunctival sensitivity testing. Loss of consciousness with respiratory arrest and seizure activity, bronchospasm, or prolonged vasomotor collapse are typical symptoms; they can, for the most part, be controlled by intravenous administration of rapidly acting barbiturates or by artificial respiration. A few fatal accidents, however, give cause for reflection, particularly since a double-blind controlled study has shown that one can forego topical anesthesia [11]. More common are aspiration pneumonias which cannot always be avoided even if the patient is placed in the left lateral decubitus position. They are a dreaded complication, particularly during emergency endoscopy, and are the reason why pharyngeal anesthesia should be avoided in this situation. There are some patients, predominantly alcoholics, who show little response to the usual premedication with narcotics, anticholinergics, barbiturates, tranquilizers, or neuroleptic analgesics; in older patients, these medications can cause transient respiratory arrest, loss of consciousness, or acute coronary insufficiency. Rigid dose schedules must be avoided at all costs; older patients frequently tolerate the examination without any premedication better than adolescents. In three-fourths of all patients, according to a study from Norway [9], an identical effect can be obtained with intravenous administration of normal saline.

Atropine should be administered prior to the examination for medicolegal reasons, even though vagovagal reflexes cannot be completely eliminated. Passage of the instrument through the esophagus and inflation of the stomach can cause arrhythmias and affect coronary perfusion. In the presence of a pre-existing abnormal ECG, transient changes such as arrhythmias, ST segment depressions, and T wave changes can occur in up to 60% of patients [6]; in rare instances, these may lead to an asystolic cardiac arrest.

All complications mentioned so far are rare, life-threatening events that require intensive therapy unless they are transient. The necessary aids for maintenance of respiration and circulation (intubation equipment, oxygen tank, suction apparatus, narcotics, antiarrhythmic agents) must be ready for use and located centrally in an endoscopy suite.

The most dreaded complication during endoscopy of the upper gastrointestinal tract is perforation of the esophagus or stomach. A perforation of the piriform sinus can be recognized during the examination by the appearance of subcutaneous emphysema in the neck. A sudden lack of distensibility of the stomach is the first clue of a perforation of this organ. In most cases the abdomen is tightly distended by the inflated air; an exploratory tap with a simple needle will cause the air to escape with a hissing noise; this obviates the radiographic demonstration of subphrenic air accumulation.

Therapy of a perforation of the esophagus depends upon the location, size, status of the wall (benign or malignant), time interval between perforation and initiation of therapy, and involvement of pleura, as well as on the patient's general condition. Some authors recommend conservative therapy for recent perforations without injury of pleura or peritoneum; however, presence of a pneumothorax, mediastinal emphysema and subcutaneous emphysema, or extravasation of water-soluble contrast media are generally considered absolute contraindications for a conservative approach.

Only in one-fourth of all perforations does the endoscopist notice any difficulties during the instrumentation. This is particularly true for gastric perforations which usually occur on the posterior wall below the cardia. In this situation one can attempt therapy with constant aspiration of gastric secretions under antibiotic prophylaxis since the acid gastric secretions are usually sterile. More reassuring for the endoscopist, however, is an active surgical approach. Perforation of the stomach by an instrument, however, is frequently unnoticed until a radiographic examination detects a clinically silent "pneumoperitoneum of unknown cause."

Following endoscopic examinations of the upper as well as the lower gastrointestinal tract, intramural air can occasionally be demonstrated radiographically. This is apparently the result of intestinal wall emphysema secondary to mucosal tears. This complication has not yet been observed following biopsy or polypectomy. Pain does not occur in this situation, and there is no danger of pneumoperitoneum. American authors [7] have repeatedly described a "pseudo-acute" abdomen following gastroscopy. In this situation insufflation of too much air, possibly aided by medication with anticholinergic drugs, leads to an acute dilatation of the stomach and small intestine with severe abdominal pain and diffuse tenderness. The radiographic diagnosis is simple; no extraluminal air can be demonstrated. Nevertheless, several patients with these symptoms have been explored because of the mistaken diagnosis of a perforation.

Bleeding following instrumentation or directed biopsy rarely becomes severe enough to require active intervention. For example, once major hemorrhage occurs after resection of a polyp or removal of a mucosal fold with a diathermy snare, it can as a rule be arrested by electrocoagulation. Finally, in the course of emergency endoscopy, recurrent bleeding from esophageal varices can be precipitated during the retroflexion maneuver for the exclusion of fundic varices. In this situation, the examination should be terminated immediately because further manipulations will only aggravate the bleeding.

During outpatient endoscopy without premedication, a spontaneous Mallory-Weiss syndrome may occasionally result from retching. Usually one finds several small mucosal tears at the transition from esophagus to cardia in conjunction with a hiatus hernia or a prominent gastroesophageal prolapse; in most cases, the bleeding will stop spontaneously after some waiting.

Bacteremia can occur during all endoscopic examinations; its course, however, is almost always clinically silent. In patients with acute leukemia, fatal *Pseudomonas* septicemias have been observed following diagnostic esophagoscopy [2]; the indication for an endoscopy, therefore, must be more restricted in these patients who already are at increased risk. Some authors recommend antibiotic prophylaxis in these high-risk patients, including in those with known valvular heart disease.

A few reports exist of incarceration of the inverted endoscope in the esophagus during retroflexion, requiring surgical removal of the instrument in some cases. The newer end-viewing panendoscopes can become retroflexed like a hairpin during introduction into the pharynx and then lodge in this form in the esophagus. If the instrument cannot be advanced into the stomach or pulled back into the pharynx, one should attempt extraction after intravenous administration of high doses of anticholinergics or glucagon. Remnants of the fourth branchial cleft, which are internal fistulae of the esophagus, so-called Compton's pockets, may fill with air during insufflation and resemble subcutaneous emphysema. They can be emptied by manual pressure without difficulty. Swelling of the submandibular gland following prolonged examination is due to transitory backup of secretions and does not require therapy.

1.4.2 Blind Biopsies

Complications during blind biopsies are rare: Hengst [3] found 36 episodes of bleeding and 2 perforations in 13,949 gastric aspiration biopsies. The situation is similar in the case of the small bowel biopsy, where perforations require surgical intervention. Occasionally, the biopsy capsule will bite into the mucosa without complete transection. In this situation, waiting until the particle has become necrotic and sloughs off will usually suffice; this may, however, take days to weeks. If the capsule cannot be removed following the hydraulic biopsy step, one should wait in any case since it can usually be removed without difficulty on the following day.

1.4.3 Retrograde Cholangiopancreatography (ERCP)

Following instillation of contrast media into the pancreatic duct system, transient hyperamylasemia occurs in about one-third of all patients, depending upon the amount of contrast media used and the pressure of instillation. This usually subsides within several days and is clinically silent. Attacks of acute pancreatitis caused by the examination are more serious; they can occur even in a "normal" pancreas, particularly when the contrast material has stained the parenchyma. The frequency of this iatrogenic pancreatitis, which cannot be prevented by prophylactic administration of aprotinin, somatostatin, calcitonin, or glucagon, is between 1%–2%.

Another dreaded complication is infection of a pancreatic pseudocyst when it has been filled with contrast medium. Since a delay in surgical intervention has frequently resulted in a fatal outcome, it is advisable to terminate the examination when a pancreatic pseudocyst is visualized and to transfer the patient to surgery for drainage of the cyst within 24 h. Our own procedure is to transfer patients who have pancreatic pseudocysts documented by ultrasound directly to the surgical department and to perform retrograde pancreatography on the day of surgery.

Dilatation of a ductal system due to outflow obstruction always predisposes to the development of a purulent inflammation. This applies particularly to stones in the common bile duct, where suppurative cholangitis with gram-negative sepsis may develop. This potential for complications can be reduced by mixing an antibiotic with the contrast medium or by direct instillation of an antibotic into the bile duct; early decompression, however, remains important. Prophylactic administration of an antibiotic, such as tetracycline as practiced by us, is controversial. The usefulness of aspiration of bile for culture and sensitivity studies is currently under study.

Rare complications that usually do not require any further therapeutic measures are bleeding from the papilla following repeated attempts at cannulation, submucosal injection of contrast medium, and loss of the metal tip of the cannula in the papilla.

1.4.4 Endoscopy of the Colon and Rectum

Rigid rectosigmoidoscopy carries the lowest risk among all endoscopic diagnostic procedures. The most dreaded complication is perforation, which almost always occurs at the transition from rectum to sigmoid. Severe pain, rapidly developing peritonitis, and symptoms of shock are unmistakable signs; proof is the subphrenic accumulation of air. The further fate of the patient depends on the time interval between perforation and surgical intervention; after an interval of 12 h, mortality already reaches 75%. Although isolated cases of successful conservative therapy have been reported, every perforation of the rectum belongs immediately in the hands of a surgeon. The same applies for perforations during colonoscopy, among which perforations due to biopsy of a diverticulum deserve special mention.

Intestinal perforation can lead to acute dyspnea due to marked abdominal distention; this can be associated with symptoms of shock requiring immediate intervention. Decompression of the pneumoperitoneum with a large-bore needle can alleviate this life-threatening condition within a few seconds [4]. While a free perforation into the abdominal cavity is immediately apparent, retroperitoneal perforations can have a largely silent course. Subcutaneous emphysema or perirenal air may point toward this complication.

Rarer complications include abscess following perforation in conjunction with passage through a stricture, incarceration of the colonoscope in a previously undetected inguinal hernia, and hematoma in the mesosigmoid caused by a forceful straightening maneuver; this manipulation can also result in rupture of the spleen.

Explosions of methane during electrosurgical procedures (coagulation, removal of polyps) have been repeatedly reported. For this reason, some examiners insufflate a noncombustible gas (CO_2) during an electrosurgical procedure. This does not appear to be necessary according to more recent studies, since no explosive gases can be detected following the intensive bowel preparation for colonoscopy [1].

Bleeding following a forceps biopsy in the course of rectosigmoidoscopy is frequent. In most instances this can be arrested by compression with a sponge soaked with thrombin or vasopressin. In addition, one may consider fulguration of the bleeding site with a coagulation electrode. Since such bleeding cannot always be controlled conservatively, forceps biopsies should not be undertaken without urgent indication if the biopsy site is beyond the reach of the operative sigmoidoscope (15–18 cm) through which the bleeding vessel can be tied with sutures, if necessary.

Cardiac arrhythmias may occur during rectosigmoidoscopy just as during endoscopy of the upper intestinal tract. In elderly patients, therefore, the customary head-down position on the rectoscopy table should be avoided. Cardiac complications, including myocardial infarction, appear to be due to postural hypotension and a reduction of the tidal volume caused by elevation of the diaphragm.

Similar to small bowel biopsies, a so-called postbiopsy syndrome may occur following biopsies of the colon; it is characterized by abdominal pain and cramping and short-lived fever. Apparently, too deep a biopsy can cause peritoneal irritation, resulting in a picture of incomplete ileus. Bacteremia has also been observed on a few occasions. It is recommended to stop oral intake for 24–48 h and to administer antibiotics directed against gram-negative organisms.

1.4.5 Blind Liver Biopsy

Harmless complications of percutaneous liver biopsy include unintentional punctures of adjacent organs such as kidney, gallbladder, colon, pancreas, adrenal gland, lung, and small intestine. Bleeding is the most common complication, with a morbidity rate of 0.29% and a mortality of 0.015% [5]. Acute hemorrhage will cause symptoms within a few hours; frequently, it will present as unusually severe abdominal pain. Even though many such hemorrhages can be controlled conservatively, cooperation with the surgeon is important for the correct timing of surgical intervention. Wildhirt [13] and other authors have mentioned late complications due to bleeding which only becomes symptomatic several days after the biopsy. More serious is bile peritonitis which presents 2–4 h after the biopsy; immediate pain suggests leakage of bile and serves as a warning sign. Further therapeutic steps depend on the clinical symptoms; active surgical intervention is preferred because of the high mortality rate.

Anglo-American authors [12] have called attention to an acute, transitory hypotension following blind liver biopsy. A sudden drop in blood pressure associated with bradycardia and epigastric pain occurs several minutes following the biopsy. It is probably mediated by vagovagal reflexes, triggered by the puncture of the pleura with the biopsy needle. Pulse and blood pressure return to normal within 20–30 min. Intraperitoneal bleeding was excluded in all cases. In doubtful situations, administration of plasma expanders is recommended.

Development of a pneumothorax, which is often incomplete, frequently goes undetected. Radiographic studies by Ortmans [8] demonstrate that this complication must be expected in 0.97% of cases, even when proper technique is used. Puncture of the pleura should always be suspected in the event of unsuccessful liver biopsy. When clinical symptoms sugest an incomplete pneumothorax, simple aspiration will often suffice; chest tubes are usually not required.

Intrahepatic arteriovenous fistulas caused by liver biopsy are rare; active intervention is required because of the potential for the development of portal hypertension. In the absence of peritoneal irritation, acute blood loss after liver biopsy suggests hemobilia due to a traumatic fistula between a hepatic artery and a bile duct.

1.4.6 Laparoscopy

Complications are much more frequently observed during laparoscopy than with any other endoscopic examination. Usually, however, these are harmless interruptions of the normal course of the procedure. Interference with the examination by adhesions or emphysema of the omentum can be overcome by detour maneuvers or by waiting. If blood or intestinal contents are aspirated during introduction of the pneumoperitoneum, the examination may be continued at a different site. If subcutaneous emphysema develops in the neck, indicating a pneumothorax or mediastinal emphysema, the procedure should be stopped, the gas removed from the peritoneal cavity, and an attempt made to let the gas escape to the highest point by placing the patient in the reverse Trendelenburg position. Cervical mediastinotomy may be required when mediastinal emphysema leads to retrosternal pressure and tightness, hyperresonance on percussion over the sternum, displacement of the apical impulse toward the left, or vena cava obstruction. In rare cases of gas emboli, sedation and pain relief in addition to oxygen administration are the mainstays of the therapeutic efforts. In the case of pulmonary gas emboli, the patient should be placed in a sitting position; in the case of cerebral gas emboli, in a head-down position. Bleeding from an organ following a biopsy can be arrested by mechanical compression with a probe, by local application of thrombin or epinephrine, or by electrocoagulation. If these measures are unsuccessful, surgical intervention becomes necessary after temporary volume expansion with colloid solution. If bile leaks from the puncture site in the liver, one should first attempt aspiration under visual control followed by coagulation. Should the leak persist, a rubber drain is placed through the trocar sleeve and left in position for 2 days. If biliary drainage does not subside after that period of time, surgical intervention is necessary.

Cardiac arrhythmias can also occur during laparoscopy, particularly during administration of CO_2 [10]. Careful patient selection will help avoid serious complications; following myocardial infarction, for instance, patients should not undergo peritoneoscopy for about 6 months. Early recognition of complications prevents serious consequences in most cases, particularly if appropriate treatment is instituted immediately. The keeping of a log of all complications, therapeutic measures, and follow-up courses is particularly useful for teaching purposes. Fortunately, serious complications during endoscopic procedures are so rare that a single individual, even with a large experience, will never encounter all possible adverse incidents.

References

1. Frühmorgen, P., Joachim, G.: Gas chromatographic analyses of intestinal gas to clarify the question of inert gas insufflation in electrosurgical endoscopy. Endoscopy *8*, 133 (1976)
2. Greene, W. H., Moody, M., Hartley, R., Effman, E., Aisner, J., Young, V. M., Wiernik, P. H.: Esophagoscopy as a source of pseudomonas aeruginosa sepsis in patients with acute leukemia: the need for sterilization of endoscopes. Gastroenterology *67*, 912–919 (1974)
3. Hengst, W.: Nil nocere! Zwischenfälle bei der Saugbiopsie des Magens. Münch. Med. Wochenschr. *45*, 2642 (1968)
4. Jacobsohn, W. Z., Levy, A.: Colonoscopic perforation: its emergency treatment. Endoscopy *8*, 15 (1976)
5. Lindner, H.: Das Risiko der perkutanen Leberbiopsie. Med. Klin. *66*, 924 (1971)
6. McEwan-Alvarado, G., Barnes, R. N., Wallace, T. I.: Electrocardiographic response to upper gastrointestinal endoscopy. Am. J. Gastroenterol. *57*, 26 (1972)
7. Moldow, R., Waye, J. D., Cohen, N.: Pseudo-acute abdomen following gastroscopy. Gastrointest. Endosc. *17*, 117 (1971)
8. Ortmans, H.: Unbemerkte Pneumothoraxentstehung nach perkutaner Leberbiopsie. Leber Magen Darm *2*, 231 (1972)
9. Peterson, H., Myren, J.: Premedication for peroral endoscopy. Two double-blind studies. Scand. J. Gastroenterol. *7*, 583 (1972)
10. Scott, D. B., Julian, D. G.: Observations on cardiac arrhythmias during laparoscopy. Brit. Med. J. *1972 I*, 411
11. Spargerg, M., Knudsen, K. B.: Is local anesthesia necessary in fibreoptic esophago-gastroscopy? A controlled study. Am. J. Dig. Dis. *12*, 1131 (1967)
12. Sullivan, S., Watson, W. C.: Acute transient hypotension as complication of percutaneous liver biopsy. Lancet *1974 I*, 389
13. Wildhirt, E.: Zur Frage der Spätkomplikation nach Leberbiopsie. Münch. Med. Wochenschr. *112*, 1234 (1970)

1.5

Gastroenterologic Biopsy (Acquisition and Processing)

K. ELSTER

The reliability of a diagnosis based on biopsy specimens depends on many factors. Diagnostic problems result not only from difficulties in interpretation and grading of the histologic pattern but frequently also from the "inadequacy" of the material. Refined technique and mastery of a method are useless without attention to detail. We will discuss these apparently trivial problems with which the pathologist must deal every day.

1.5.1 Acquisition of Material

The methodology section describes "how" one obtains material by forceps biopsy. The question of "where" or "from where" the material has been obtained is of immediate importance to the endoscopist as well as the pathologist. An example from daily practice will demonstrate the uncertainty with which this question may be answered.

Two particles of gastric mucosa are submitted without stating the biopsy site, with the following simple notation, "gastric biopsy with question of atrophic gastritis." Both specimens show antral mucosa with low-grade superficial gastritis. Although this "result" could stimulate a whole series of clinical interpretations, only two rhetorical questions will be asked that are intended to be provocative

1) How does the endoscopist interpret this histologic diagnosis?
2) Should one not consider the entire examination as unsatisfactory?

This inadequate performance leads to a description of the following prerequisites and conclusions.

1.5.1.1 Diagnosis of Gastritis

In a rather high percent of cases, gastritis is not a diffuse process equally developed throughout the entire stomach, particularly with regard to its severity. This has been proven by obtaining biopsies along the lesser and greater curvatures, with removal of 12 particles at nearly equal intervals [2]. This method, justifiably considered too laborious by many examiners, is probably not necessary for the routine diagnostic evaluation, particularly since its results are of no therapeutic consequence. Two particles from the antrum and two from the body, preferably from the anterior wall toward the greater curvature, should be sufficient to permit a survey of the spectrum of gastritis.

The specimens from the two gastric regions with different mucosal structure, however, must be submitted separately, i.e., in two separate bottles. If the hospital has a pathologist so that mailing is not required, it will suffice to place the biopsy specimens on appropriately marked strips of paper and to place the loaded strips carefully in the formalin solution, which will save one bottle (the two-bottle method, of course, is more reliable).

This "cumbersome procedure" is necessary because atrophic gastritis of the mucosa of the gastric body is characterized by transformation of the fundic glands, whose main characteristics are the chief and parietal cells, into mucoid glands of the antral type. Absence of fundic glands in the specimens may indicate atrophic gastritis of the mucosa of the gastric body; however, it is also possible that only antral mucosa was obtained (for instance, in the case of a proximal displacement of the border between the antrum and body). This finding would then have to be interpreted as superficial gastritis of the antral mucosa.

The need to submit the specimens in separate bottles is underscored by a situation of diagnostic as well as therapeutic importance, where nearly normal antral mucosa exists in the presence of advanced chronic atrophic gastritis in the body, such as in pernicious anemia. The "mixing" of the particles can result in misinterpretation, since antral mucosa close to the pylorus frequently shows intestinal metaplasia, which in this particular location should only be considered as a local variant of the mucosa. Assignment of this intestinal metaplasia to the mucosa of the body may result in the wrong diagnosis of chronic atrophic gastritis.

1.5.1.2 Hyperplasias

The diagnosis of mucosal hyperplasia requires that the particles obtained are suitable for quantitative interpretation. The main examples of diffuse hyperplasia are the glandular type of the Zollinger-Ellison syndrome and the foveolar type of Menetrier's disease. The biopsy particles must be of sufficient size for the mucosal and cut surfaces to be clearly recognizable during the imbedding in paraffin. This will guarantee a precisely vertical cutting plane. Mucosal thickness can be determined only in those specimens that show sharp contours of the gastric pits and crests on the surface, whose glandular bodies show evenly stretched glandular tubules that can be surveyed in their entire length, and in which the base consists of muscularis mucosae. In this situation, the measurable entity, i.e., the thickness in millimeters, is the objective basis of the evaluation. It is admittedly difficult to obtain these sharply contoured particles with a forceps, and an aspiration biopsy will usually be superior. One can overcome this disadvantage by obtaining a large number of particles and also by removing tissue in a systematic fashion to document the diffuse hyperplasia present in the Zollinger-Ellison syndrome. In concrete terms, this means that in cases where Zollinger-Ellison syndrome is suspected, multiple particles should be removed between the antrum and the fundus close to the cardia, at about equal intervals. One can thereby demonstrate the border between body and antrum which may be displaced distally in diffuse hyperplasia. Of course, the biopsy particles will have to be submitted in several bottles with precise statements about their sites of origin. One should forego the counting of parietal cells, since not every pathologist is a mathematician. With biopsy particles, this will not yield any reliable results anyway and merely amounts to a symbolic act.

In Menetrier's disease, mucosal particles should be removed from the crests of the folds as well as from the valleys since focal hyperplasia may be present in the latter areas also.

Development of the snare biopsy, a method originally restricted to polypectomy, has provided another means of demonstrating mucosal hyperplasia morphologically. In large particle biopsies [3], the base of the cut usually lies in the submucosa so that the entire height or width of the mucosa is enclosed; in addition, the opportunity exists to discover submucosal changes. The particles, which can be as large as a bean, should be spread on a strip of paper or cardboard prior to fixation to avoid warping or coiling. Particles and paper strips have to be placed immediately into formalin-containing bottles of sufficient size.

1.5.1.3 Localized Processes

For the diagnostic evaluation of localized processes by biopsy, one should apply the following basic rule: "as much as possible and from as many areas as possible." In principle, six to ten particles should be removed because frequently one finds changes representative of a localized process in only one or two biopsy particles. "Multiple sites" means that one should pay attention to variability in the structure within the local lesion. This not only applies to ulcerative processes but also to flat polypoid lesions. The flat recess that appears as an ulcer crater should not be "off limits"; particularly in the fairly common type IIc of early carcinoma, the characteristic changes are found in the "ulcer base." To define the peripheral extension of a suspected cancerous lesion, biopsies should also be obtained from adjacent areas. The answer to this important question, however, can only be given if these particles are submitted separately with the appropriate topographic identification. Identical ground rules apply to flat polypoid lesions.

For histologic classification and diagnosis of "true" polyps, biopsy from the tip, base, and stalk was customary. This approach is no longer justified since the diagnosis can be made with greater accuracy by removal of the entire polyp with a snare. Biopsy from the stalk and the base to discover possible infiltrative growth of a carcinoma, in analogy to the polypoid adenomas of the colon, is not applicable to gastric polyps. For the epithelial gastric polyps, generally an "either/or" decision has to be made. If a biopsy from the apex shows focal hyperplasia with highly differentiated epithelial cells, one is dealing either with a hyperplastic polyp (focal hyperplasia) or with an adenomatous, mixed form of a hyperplastic polyp. Both kinds of polyp are benign and show no tendency for malignant degeneration. On the other hand, if one finds "suspicious" atypia of the epithelium, one may be dealing with a precancerous lesion, such as glandular neck proliferation with cellular atypia (borderline lesion) or even with an early carcinoma type I or IIa. In the first situation, where benign epithelial polyps are demonstrated, polypectomy would be the preferred course of action. In the latter case, i.e., in the case of a suspected early carcinoma type I or IIa, surgical intervention is unavoidable [4].

The same general rules apply for biopsy of localized processes in the colon. Single as well as multiple biopsies from a polyp will provide diagnostic results only in the case of a benign hyperplastic polyp with a characteristic surface structure. The question of "malignant degeneration" of a polypoid adenoma cannot be answered on the basis of incomplete excision, i.e., biopsy. Cellular atypia is an obligatory characteristic of these adenomatous polyps. The transition to carcinoma is characterized by infiltrating growth by these atypical glands into the submucosa and, thus, by penetration of the muscularis mucosae. In assessing the biologic nature of these adenomatous polyps, an answer to the question of "benign" or "malignant" requires a completely excised specimen with broad segments of the base of the polyp. As a practical consequence, the first diagnostic step is polypectomy. Of course, the diagnosis of polypoid or ulcerating carcinoma can also be made on the basis of one or two representative specimens. The pathologist should always be informed about the location, size, and structure of the lesion and whether it has a pedicle or a broad base; this information may be of decisive importance for the interpretation of the histologic findings, particularly in the case of adenomatous polyps.

Generalized colonic disorders, such as ulcerative colitis and Crohn's disease, may also be considered histologically as "localized processes." Particularly in the latter situation, the mucosal lesions can be definitely focal so that one should never be satisfied with one or two particles. Without knowledge of the clinical picture one can only expect a descriptive histologic diagnosis. Rectal biopsies for the diagnosis of amyloidosis should, if at all possible, contain submucosa since one can expect deposits of amyloid with greater frequency in this area due to its higher vascularity.

1.5.2 Processing of Biopsy Material

The processing of material is not only the task of the pathologist. It starts with the excision, i.e., with the transfer of the biopsy specimens to the fixative solution. For small biopsy particles, a 4% formalin solution is satisfactory. Immediately upon removal, the biopsy specimen has to be immersed in the solution, rather than adding the fixative to the jar later. The particle must "float" and not stick to the wall. Flasks with tapered bottoms are unsuitable, particularly for larger specimens, such as resected polyps or large fold biopsies, since the particles frequently stick to the tapered end and can only be removed with sharp objects. The number and nature of the specimens should be noted on the label of the bottle, as well as on the referral slip. Experience, it should be stressed, teaches that the labels must be identical. The referral slips, which should bear the address of the referring physician as well as that of the patient, are not suitable as immediate wrapping material for the formalin-filled bottles. A few drops of formalin are sufficient to make such a document illegible.

1.5.2.1 Information on Clinical Data and Findings

The pathologist's interest in history and clinical findings should not be interpreted by the clinician as a "weakness." The interpretation of the histologic findings in many cases will depend decisively upon knowledge of the macroscopic or endoscopic findings. It is "old-fashioned" to think that these subjective data will cloud the objective judgment of the pathologist.

1.5.2.2 Documentation of Early Carcinoma of the Stomach

Diagnostic efforts to clarify the nature of localized processes are directed particularly at the detection of early carcinoma of the stomach. Diagnosis of this type of carcinoma, characterized by its good prognosis, can only be proven in a resected stomach, i.e., one must define the extent of the carcinoma on the surface and, particularly, in its depth. This rather laborious and time-consuming examination can only be successful if the surgical specimen arrives in the hands of the pathologist in a state in which even minor changes in the mucosal profile can be recognized. This is impossible if the resected stomach is stuffed into the "usual" jar with formalin poured over it. This preparation, deformed by the fixation process, does not allow the careful examination required. The pathologist, therefore, has to demand, not only recommend, the following procedure:

1) The resected specimen should be opened along the greater curvature, unless the lesion is situated there.
2) The opened specimen should be loosely attached to cardboard with pins (no stretching!).
3) The specimen should be fixed in a large jar (cardboard on top, surface of stomach facing downward, submerged in the fluid), containing 10% formalin, for about 1½ days.
4) The specimen, including the cardboard, should be placed in a cellophane or plastic bag and sealed tightly (no prior rinsing).
5) The plastic bag should be placed in a padded envelope (as used for mailing of books) and mailed in this form.

According to Büchner [1], adherence to pragmatism constitutes a misunderstanding of the role of science. One should accept this with a grain of salt. We want to emphasize the importance of this grain of salt; neither the artist nor the scientist can function without craftsman-like skills.

References

1. Büchner, F.: Allgemeine und Spezielle Pathologie. Dtsch. Med. Wochenschr. *83*, 1885–1887 (1958)
2. Ottenjann, R., Rösch, W., Elster, K.: Ist die Gastritis ein diffuser Prozeß? Klin. Wochenschr. *49*, 27–31 (1971)
3. Ottenjann, R., Lux, G., Henke, M., Strauch, M.: Big Particle Biopsy. Endoscopy *5*, 139–143 (1973)
4. Rösch, W., Elster, K.: Gastrointestinale Präkanzerosen. Baden-Baden: Witzstock 1977

1.6

Gastroenterologic Cytology (Acquisition and Processing)

S. WEIDENHILLER

Gastroenterologic cytology is a search for tumor cells in brushings from the mucosal surfaces, in the sediment of duodenal secretions and ascitic fluid, and in material aspirated from suspected malignant tumors [8].

1.6.1 Endoscopic Brush Cytology

Instruments. Endoscopic scrapings are obtained with cytology brushes that fit the respective endoscopes as marketed by the manufacturers. Some brushes come with plastic tubes; the brush can be retracted into the tip of the tube after the scraping so that withdrawal through the instrument channel is possible without loss of material (Fig. 1).

Patient Preparation and Postprocedure Care. These are determined by the endoscopic procedure.

Technique. This can be learned easily; however, the scraping must be done carefully. The superficial epithelial layers are lifted from an endoscopically suspicious area by a to-and-fro movement of the brush, which is pressed tightly against the mucosa. The movements of the brush are coordinated with corresponding movements of the endoscope in such a way that the entire lesion and the surrounding area are sampled (Fig. 2). Brush and plastic tube are then pulled back through the instrument channel. The

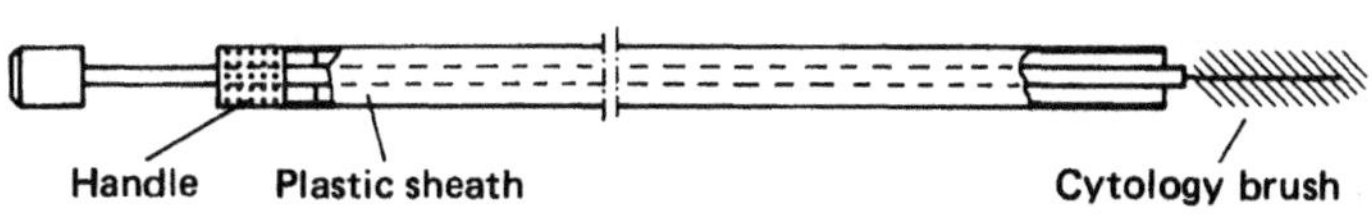

Fig. 1. Cytology brush with sheath and handle.

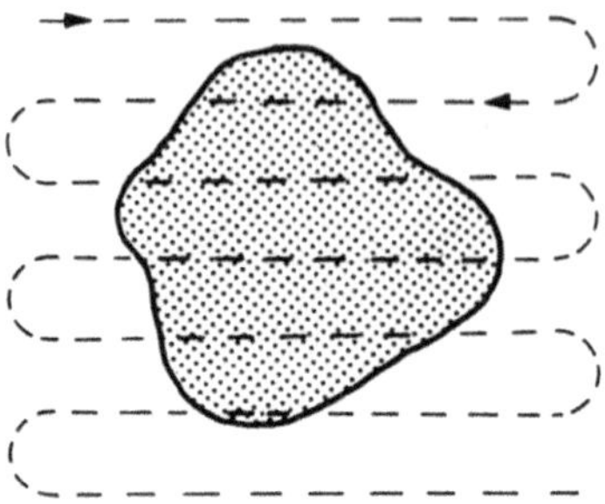

Fig. 2. Use of the cytology brush: movement of the brush across a suspicious lesion and the adjacent area.

brushing itself can be obtained at any time during the endoscopic examination. Brushes without the plastic tube can also be withdrawn through the instrument channel. Because a large amount of scraped material will be retained in the channel, the procedure should be repeated once or twice. An alternative is to obtain the brushing at the end of the endoscopic examination and to withdraw the brush into the tip of the instrument channel (Fig. 3) to avoid stripping of the material during withdrawal of the endoscope.

The cell material must be processed immediately, up to and including fixation, to obtain useable cytologic preparations (Fig. 4). After the brush has been rinsed in a few milliliters of normal saline, which is most easily done in a test tube, the cell suspensions are centrifuged for 5–8 min at 3000 rpm, the supernatant is decanted, and the sediment spread with a cotton tip or a plastic loop. Fixation is best accomplished with a spray fixative (Merko-Fix, Adams Spray-Cyte) according to the manufacturer's instructions. Other procedures can also be used (a 1:1 mixture of 96% alcohol and ether, duration 20 min; glycerol-96% alcohol, 1:4, duration 20 min). The slides are then stained according to Papanicolaou (for details see references [4–5]). The slides treated with the spray fixative are also suitable for mailing to cytology institutes. Slides with a frosted end, on which the name of the patient and the source of the material can be written with pencil, are recommended. The preliminary macroscopic diagnosis should be noted on the referral slip. Other staining techniques can be used but are not required. They give poorer results than the Papanicolaou stain in gastroenterologic brush cytology and should be used only if the latter is not available.

Pappenheim stain: the material is smeared on the slide and air-dried.

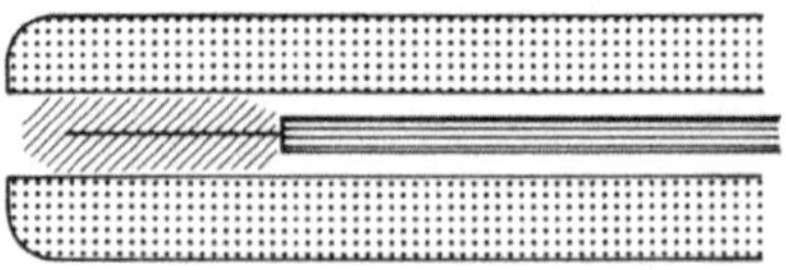

Fig. 3. Retraction of the cytology brush without plastic sheath into instrumentation channel after lesion has been brushed.

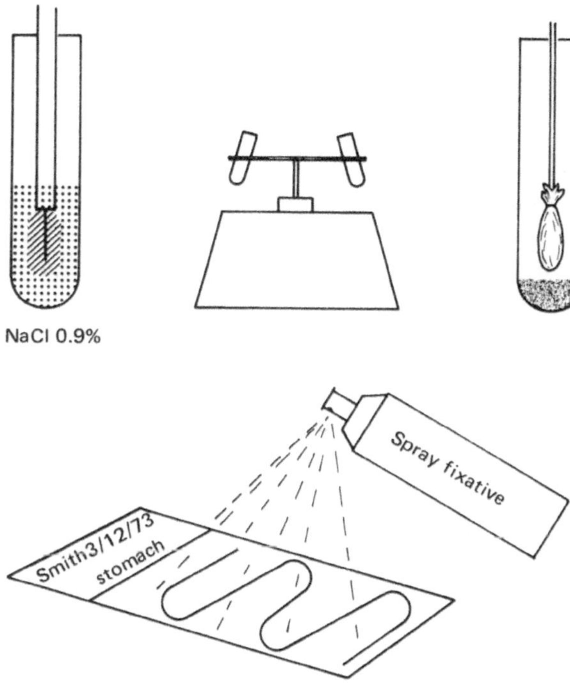

Fig. 4. Preparation of cytology specimen: washing the cytology brush, centrifugation, smear, and fixation.

Thereafter, the standard staining technique is used (literature in [2]). This staining technique has the frequent disadvantage that transparency of the preparations is reduced because mucus, debris, and fibrin stain intensively and may cover the cell clusters. Similarly, cell clusters consisting of several layers cannot be evaluated due to superimposition of individual cells. On the other hand, structures of individual cells can be identified well with this staining technique.

Reis stain (for details see reference [4]): fixation of the moist specimen with a mixture of alcohol and ether (ether-96% alcohol, 1:1), stain with a 1% solution of safranine for 2–3 min, differentiate with absolute alcohol until no further clouds of color are removed, rinse with distilled water, counterstain for 10 min with a May-Grünwald-Giemsa solution (1 ml May-Grünwald solution, 5 drops Giemsa stock solution, 5 ml distilled water), rinse, and finally, air-dry. This stain yields sufficiently transparent preparations with good resolution of detail and can be recommended as a substitute if the Papanicolaou stain is not available.

Indications. Brushings should be obtained from all lesions seen during endoscopy of the esophagus, stomach, small intestine, and colon in which a malignant process cannot be excluded with certainty.

Contraindications and Complications. These correspond to those of the endoscopic examination.

1.6.2 Cytology of Duodenal Aspirates

Indications. Suspected malignant tumors of the pancreas, the biliary tree, or the duodenum.

1.6.2.1 Cytology Obtained by Duodenal Intubation

Instruments, Preparation, Postprocedure Care, Contraindications, and Complications. These correspond to those of the pancreozymin-secretin test for the evaluation of exocrine pancreas function [1]. Both procedures should always be performed simultaneously.

Technique. Altogether, seven collections are examined: one sample of basal secretion and three samples each of duodenal secretions stimulated by secretin and pancreozymin. The stimulated secretions are collected in 10-min fractions. After removal of the portion required for chemical determinations, the entire remaining aspirate is centrifuged (for about 5–8 min at 3000 rpm). The sediment is used to prepare five smears, of which four are stained according to Papanicolaou following wet fixation [4,5] and one according to Pappenheim after air-drying [2] (details see Sect. 1.6.1). The remainder of the sediment is fixed in 10% formalin and mailed for examination by the cell block method.

Immediate processing of the duodenal aspirate is absolutely necessary to avoid destruction of the cells which occurs very rapidly in this medium. Two methods have been described to prevent cytolysis; according to our own experience, however, their effectiveness does not justify the effort: (a) trapping of the duodenal secretions in tubes that contain about 5 ml of a mixture of Trasylol and 0.2 ml EDTA (Titriplex III—ethylene diamine tetra-acetate) (literature in [4]) or (b) storage of the secretions in ice-cold containers.

1.6.2.2 Aspiration of Secretions by Endoscopy

Instruments, Preparation, Postprocedure Care, Contraindications, and Complications. These correspond to those of postbulbar duodenoscopy (p. 74).

Technique. When the papilla of Vater is inspected during duodenoscopy, secretin is injected prior to any other manipulations (1 unit/kg body weight) and the secretions are aspirated from the papilla with a syringe,

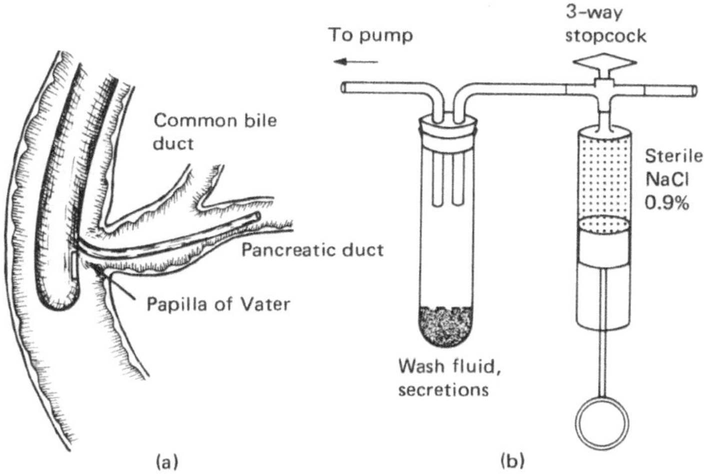

Fig. 5. Intubation of pancreatic duct (a); apparatus for flushing the duct and for aspiration of secretions (b).

through the plastic cannula normally used for cannulation. Selective endoscopic retrograde cannulation of the ducts (pancreatic duct, common bile duct) can also be combined with acquisition of material for cytology.

Before X-ray contrast material is instilled, the ampulla of Vater or, preferably, the desired ductal system is cannulated (Fig. 5). The catheter is connected via a three-way stopcock, either to a 10-cc syringe containing sterile saline, or to a test tube serving as a trap for the secretions. A suction pump or 20-cc syringe is connected to this secretion trap, 1–2 cc of saline are instilled, transient negative pressure is applied, and the injected fluid trapped in the test tube. This procedure is repeated about eight to ten times. Subsequently, secretin (1 unit/kg body weight) is again given intravenously, and the draining secretions are aspirated for about 15–20 min by intermittent low suction. The material is processed as described for the cytology of duodenal secretions (Sect. 1.6.2.1).

1.6.3 Fine Needle Aspiration

1.6.3.1 Fine Needle Aspiration of Abdominal Organs Under Ultrasound Control

Instruments. Required are an ultrasound apparatus with two-dimensional recording mode (e.g., Vidoson apparatus, Siemens Company, Erlangen), aspiration needles with an external diameter of 0.7–0.8 mm and a length of 2–12 cm (Storz Company, Tuttlingen), and 10- or 20-cc syringes for aspiration. Detailed descriptions of the technique of ultrasound examination are available [3].

Patient Preparation. Coagulation panel (prothrombin time, partial thromboplastin time, platelet count); for aspiration of the liver, bilirubin and alkaline phosphatase; for renal aspiration, an intravenous pyelogram.

Postprocedure Care. Observation for 24 h to exclude bleeding by monitoring pulse and blood pressure; another ultrasound study if bleeding is suspected.

Technique. Puncture site and direction of the needle are determined by the sonographic image. The distance of the lesion from the skin is measured on the projection screen and marked on the cannula with either a tape or a guard. After disinfection and local anesthesia of the puncture site, the cannula is advanced to the predetermined depth of penetration. By combining suction with gentle to-and-fro movement of the cannula, material is aspirated from the suspicious site over a period of 0.5–1.0 s; the suction is then released and the cannula removed. The aspirated material is transferred to a slide with a frosted end by repeated gentle flushing of the cannula with air. It is then spread by applying very gentle pressure with the aspiration cannula or by using a cover slip. Large admixtures of blood can be removed gently with blotting paper. After drying in air, the slides, carrying the patient's name, are stained according to Pappenheim [2].

Indications. Possible tumors observed by ultrasound in the liver, the pancreas, and in the abdominal wall. In the case of renal tumors, fine needle aspiration should be performed only after consultation with the urologist.

Contraindications. Marked clotting abnormalities, severe obstructive jaundice.

Complications. Bleeding; in the presence of icterus, bile peritonitis.

1.6.3.2 Fine Needle Aspiration During Laparoscopy

Indications. Indications exist only if removal of biopsy material for histologic examination is impossible, particularly in cases of liver metastases and pancreatic tumors.

Instruments, Patient Preparation, Postprocedure Care, Technique, Contraindications, and Complications. As with fine needle aspiration under ultrasound control (Sec. 1.6.3.1).

References

1. Barthelheimer, H.: In Klinische Gastroenterologie. Demling, L. (Ed.). Stuttgart: Thieme 1973
2. Begemann, H., Harwerth, H. G.: Praktische Hämotologie. Stuttgart: Thieme 1970

3. ENGELHART, G. J., BLAUENSTEIN, U. W.: Ultraschalldiagnostik am Oberbauch. Stuttgart, New York: Schattauer 1972
4. HENNING, N., WITTE, S.: Atlas der gastroenterologischen Cytodiagnostik. Stuttgart: Thieme 1968
5. KOSS, G.: Diagnostic Cytology. Philadelphia, Toronto: Lippincott 1968
6. LUTZ, H.: Ultraschalldiagnostik (B-Scan) in der Inneren Medizin. Berlin, Heidleberg, New York: Springer 1978
7. LUTZ, H., WEIDENHILLER, S., RETTENMAIER, G.: Ultraschallgezielte Feinnadelbiopsie der Leber. Schweiz. Med. Wochenschr. *103*, 1030 (1973)
8. WITTE, S.: In: Gastroenterologische Endoskopie, Biopsie und Zytologie. OTTENJANN, R., ELSTER, K., WITTE, S. (Ed.). Stuttgart: Thieme 1970

2

Special Section

2.1 Esophagogastroduodenoscopy

W. RÖSCH

Until a few years ago, endoscopy of the esophagus and stomach was limited to answering specific questions raised by a preceding radiographic examination. The development of fully flexible fiberendoscopes that can be controlled externally and, in particular, the construction of end-viewing optical systems have changed the indications for esophagogastroduodenoscopy completely. Since clinical everyday practice demonstrates that one must anticipate multiple abnormalities in 16% of all patients, the inspection of the entire upper intestinal tract in one procedure, including the postbulbar duodenum, is now endoscopic routine. In many places it is not only used for endoscopic biopsy verification of suspected abnormalities but, more importantly, for the diagnostic evaluation of ill-defined and atypical upper abdominal complaints.

2.1.1 Instruments

A multitude of instruments is available for endoscopic diagnostic studies of the upper digestive tract. The choice of the manufacturer will partly depend on the basic equipment already available, particularly the light sources, and partly on the customer service offered. Among the fiberoptic instruments, the American and Japanese products continue to be technically superior.

Despite their outstanding image quality, the rigid and semirigid instruments have largely gone out of fashion because the risk of complications is ten times higher than with comparable flexible models. The physician who has used a rigid esophagoscope, however, will be reluctant to do without this instrument in certain situations.

The short flexible esophagoscopes, whose extended modifications allowed inspection of portions of the stomach, have been made superfluous by the 120-cm long end-viewing instruments.

The role of the side-viewing gastroscopes has also been diminished, perhaps unduly so, by the availability of extremely flexible end-viewing esophagogastroduodenoscopes. For limited diagnostic evaluation of the stomach, such as endoscopic biopsy and follow-up of an ulcer at the incisura, or of a lesion on the posterior wall below the cardia, they remain unsurpassed and ideally suited for the beginner who may still have some difficulty in manipulating the end-viewing instruments. Esophagogastroduodenoscopes with end-viewing optics and a tip flexible in two planes should be the standard instruments of an endoscopy section. Almost all desired information can be obtained by their use; they are distinctly superior to the old gastroscopes because of their built-in flushing and suction devices.

Side-viewing duodenoscopes, as used for the retrograde cannulation of ductal systems, are rarely necessary for complete inspection of a scarred duodenal bulb or of the postbulbar duodenum. A so-called tiltable lens was recently developed for the same purpose, which allows changing from an end-viewing to a side-viewing position (Figs. 1–4).

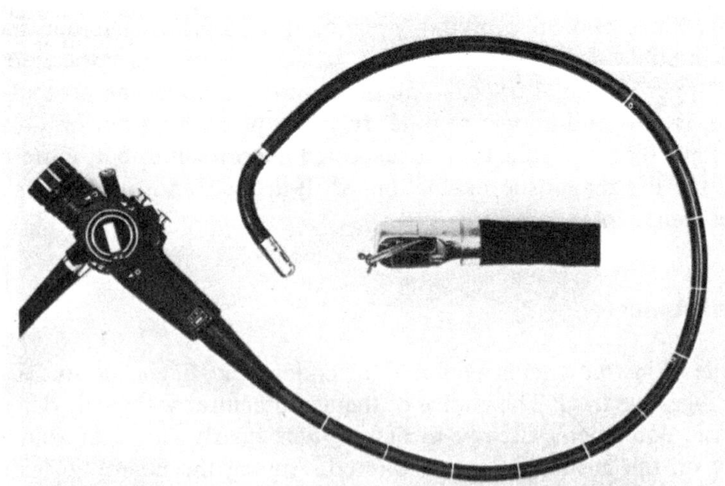

Fig. 1. Side-viewing endoscope Olympus GF-B2.

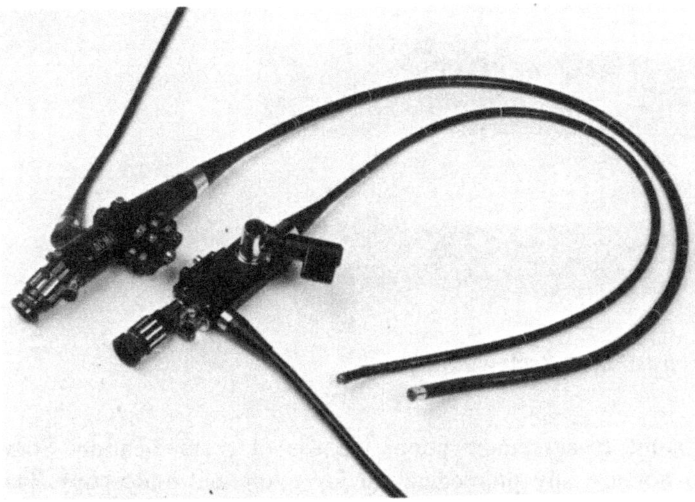

Fig. 2. End-viewing endoscopes ACMI TX-8 and FX-7.

2.1.2 Patient Preparation

Every endoscopic examination of the upper alimentary tract with the exception, of course, of emergency procedures should be preceded by a radiographic study. This is particularly necessary for examinations with side-viewing instruments that do not allow inspection of the esophagus. Prothrombin time, partial thromboplastin time, and platelet count should be determined to exclude a bleeding diathesis. While an electrocardiogram to exclude cardiac arrhythmias, chest X-ray for the exclusion of aortic aneurysm, and blood typing are not absolutely necessary, these examinations will already have been done during the work-up of many patients. It is self-evident that only a fasting patient can be examined with optimal results. Informed consent should have been obtained.

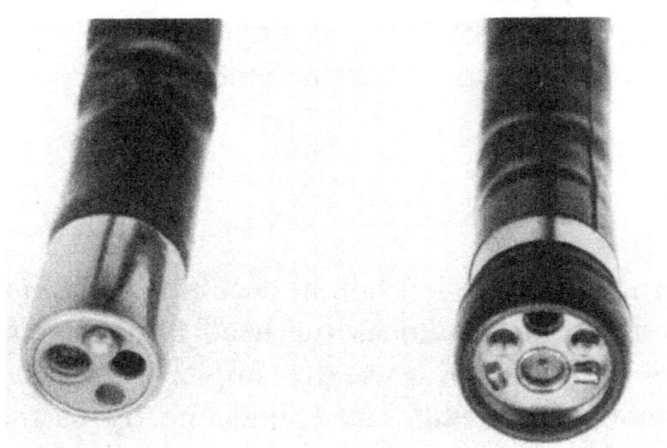

Fig. 3. Tips of instruments (end-viewing).

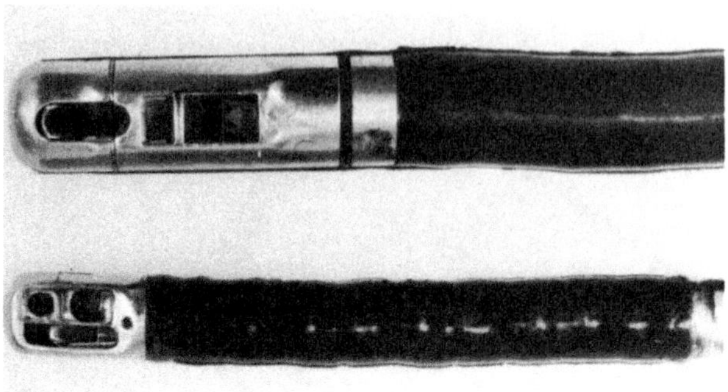

Fig. 4. Tips of instruments (side-viewing).

There is some disagreement about the use of premedication. Some institutions do not use any premedication for outpatient endoscopy. Our experience leads us to recommend the following policy: The patient receives 0.5 mg of atropine sulfate and 10 mg Vesprin (triflupromazine), IM, 30 min prior to the examination. Before introduction of the instrument, the patient is given 20 cc of a defoaming agent to drink [Mylicor (dimethylpolysiloxane)]; subsequently, the pharynx is anesthesized with a Novesine spray (oxybuprocaine). Meperidin, 50–100 mg IV, creates ideal conditions for the examination; this is not achieved to an equal degree by other tranquilizers (Valium, 10 mg, IV). Dentures must be removed prior to the examination.

2.1.3 Postprocedure Care

Special postprocedure care following esophagogastroduodenoscopy is not required. Even after multiple biopsies, bleeding need not be anticipated. The patient should be kept fasting for 1–2 h, however, because of the danger of aspiration following pharyngeal anesthesia. Moreover, the premedication will be effective for several hours and may impair the patient's judgment; this is an important consideration with outpatients.

2.1.4 Technique

We prefer to introduce the instrument in the left lateral decubitus position; if rigid esophagoscopes are used, an aid should fix the head firmly in extreme dorsal extension. For fiber endoscopy it is usually simpler if the head is flexed anteriorly. The left hand of the examiner splints the tip of the instrument between index and middle fingers and, at the same time, pushes

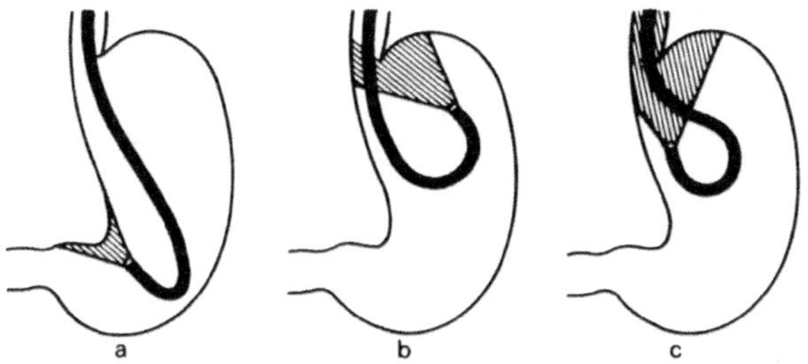

Fig. 5, a–c. Retroflexion with end-viewing optics; **a** in antrum for inspection of the incisura; **b** retroflexion over the greater curvature; **c** retroflexion over the lesser curvature.

the back of the tongue anteriorly, while the right hand advances the instruments. The experienced examiner can frequently do without the aid of the left hand and introduces the instrument as if it were a gastric tube. Deep inspiration and swallowing during passage of the instrument through the upper esophageal sphincter will facilitate the introduction. If elastic resistance is encountered at about 15 cm distance, the instrument has deviated into the left or right piriform sinus.

Further advance into the esophagus must occur under direct vision, particularly during passage of the gastroesophageal junction. For the combined examination of esophagus, stomach, and duodenum, the instrument is rapidly advanced into the duodenum through the partially inflated stomach. The actual examination occurs as the instrument is withdrawn. Passage through the pylorus is occasionally somewhat difficult; it will always be successful if one uses end-viewing optics and places the pyloric opening in the center of the visual field.

A retroflexion maneuver should be performed in the antrum to inspect the incisura angularis from below if the instrument tip can be deflected by 180°. As during the "high inversion," the tip is maximally flexed to form a U shape. For inspection of the cardia, the same maneuver is performed in the center of the body, along the lesser and the greater curvature, so that the cardia can be inspected from all sides (Fig. 5). With side-viewing instruments, the inversion maneuver is possible only along the greater curvature because the relatively long tip can only be angled by 90°. Therefore, the large folds of the greater curvature must be visualized first; the instrument is then flexed into a J shape and advanced along the greater curvature toward the dome of the fundus, until the cardia is visualized (Fig. 6). The further course of the examination is depicted in Fig. 7.

Deposits of mucus on the mucosa can usually be flushed off with a well-aimed water jet. If no spontaneous peristalsis occurs or if localized infiltration of the wall is suspected, metoclopramide (Reglan) may be

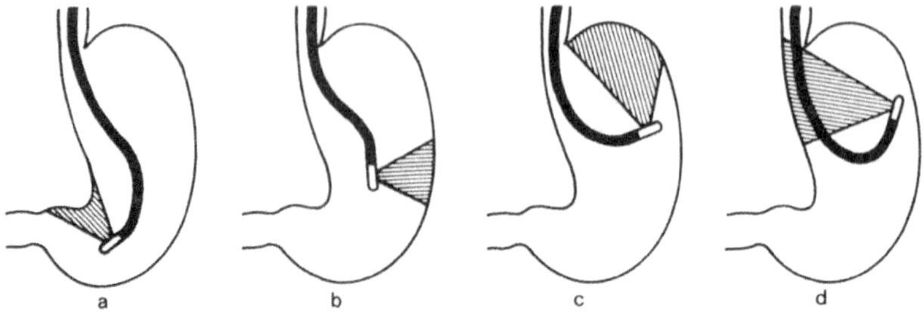

Fig. 6, a–d. Retroflexion with side-viewing instrument; **a** search for incisura; **b** turning of the instrument with view of the greater curvature; **c** advancing of the instrument along the greater curvature; **d** final position with view of the cardia.

given intravenously. For optimal evaluation of the duodenal bulb, which can only be incompletely inflated, administration of anticholinergics or of glucagon (0.4–1.0 mg) intravenously is recommended.

To obtain representative mucosal particles, the biopsy forceps should be pushed firmly into the tissue until it bends slightly. The forceps will then usually grasp the entire thickness of the mucosa to the depth of the muscularis mucosae. In the presence of localized mucosal changes, as many pieces of tissue as possible should be obtained. A minimum of six specimens is recommended.

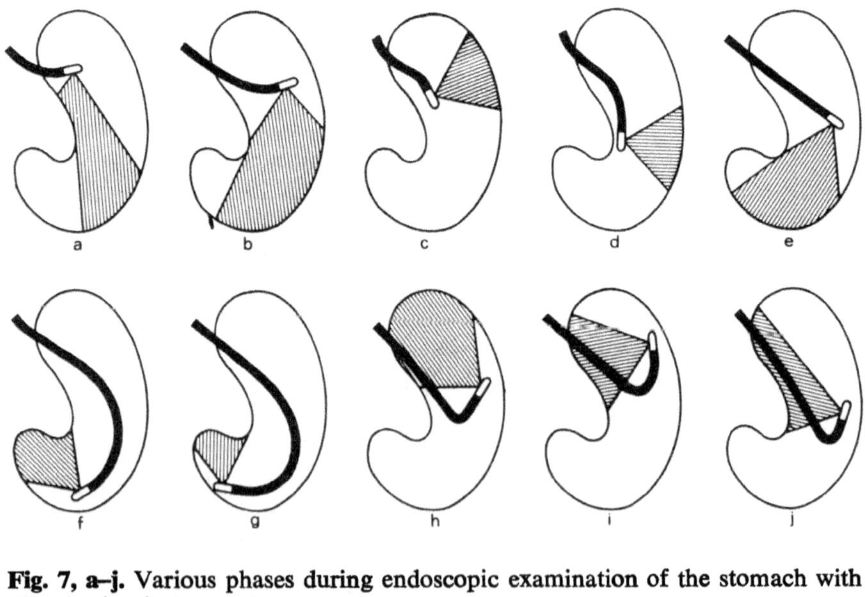

Fig. 7, a–j. Various phases during endoscopic examination of the stomach with side-viewing instrument.

Endoscopic chromography of the border between the antrum and body is not widely used because it is rather cumbersome and of little clinical relevance. Only limited experience is available with the so-called dye-scattering method, in which methylene blue or cardio-green is sprayed through a Teflon tube onto the mucosa to make subtle differences in the mucosal surface more apparent [3].

Special diagnostic methods and endoscopic therapeutic procedures in the upper digestive tract will be described in a separate section (p. 111).

2.1.5 Indications

Endoscopic examination of the upper digestive tract aims to confirm by biopsy radiographically suspected malignancies, to localize sources of bleeding, and to obtain additional information in cases with negative radiographic studies.

An endoscopic evaluation of the esophagus is always indicated when dysphagia persists for longer than 2 weeks. A change in the mucosal profile seen on X ray requires confirmation by histology and cytology; the "score rate" in the presence of carcinoma is about 60% with rigid instruments, while it approaches 100% with fiber endoscopes when cytologic material is obtained simultaneously [6]. The differentiation between a squamous cell carcinoma and a carcinoma of the cardia extending into the esophagus is important for planning the therapeutic approach. While the diagnosis of a diaphragmatic hernia can be accomplished more easily and, probably, more reliably by radiography, the consequences of an incompetent lower esophageal sphincter in the presence of a hiatus hernia can be demonstrated only by endoscopy. Esophageal varices seen during radiographic evaluation will also be seen by endoscopy. The endoscopist will, in addition, find varices in 25%–60% of cases that escaped detection during routine radiographic study [7]. Endoscopic evaluation of the esophagus, therefore, is part of the "obligatory work-up" of all patients with chronic liver disease.

Early recognition of malignant changes is the aim of the endoscopic evaluation of the stomach. For this purpose, it is essential to remove tissue under direct vision from all localized mucosal lesions; of particular importance are gastric ulcers or lesions similar in appearance to gastric ulcers. Small carcinomas can be detected only by systematic biopsy of all gastric ulcers. Giant gastric folds can have quite variable histologic features, ranging from benign hyperplasias to systemic illnesses. Mucosal erosions, particularly in the antrum, are frequently missed or misinterpreted on radiographic examination, and endoscopy is used to exclude the possibility of malignancy. Gastric polyps are removed completely with a diathermy snare and are further processed by serial sections to exclude a polypoid carcinoma.

A detailed inspection of the duodenal bulb will frequently demonstrate ulcers that have escaped radiographic detection [4]. Although malignancies in the duodenal bulb and the postbulbar duodenum are extremely rare, duodenoscopy will help to free many patients from the stigma of having "neurotic" gastrointestinal complaints. Erosive changes in the bulb, scars from previous bulbar ulcers, and high-grade deformities of the bulb due to scar formation may help explain complaints suggesting a duodenal ulcer that is not seen on X-ray or during endoscopy [2]. The pylorus can be visualized only with an end-viewing instrument; this area is a "blind spot" for side-viewing optics. Postbulbar ulcers are relatively rare. They should be specifically searched for in the presence of appropriate clinical symptoms.

The postoperative stomach is a special indication for endoscopic evaluation because its pockets and niches are frequently confusing to the radiologist. Some centers even forego a prior radiographic examination. Practically all anastomotic ulcers can be demonstrated with end- and side-viewing optics. The afferent and efferent loops should be intubated and inspected for peptic lesions. Occasionally, remaining antral mucosa in the blind duodenal stump can be identified by biopsy as a cause of an anastomotic ulcer [5]. Nonabsorbable suture material can be removed during the examination with the biopsy forceps or a special diathermy probe [1]. The early recognition of recurrent gastric carcinoma and of a carcinoma newly developing in the gastric remnant are two special aims of endoscopy in the patient with prior gastric surgery (see also Sect. 2.2).

Emergency esophagogastroduodenoscopy has become of decisive importance for identification of the sites of acute gastrointestinal bleeding. Endoscopy is performed after the cardiovascular system has been stabilized, without preceding X-ray examination, premedication, or pharyngeal anesthesia (to avoid aspiration pneumonia); even gastric lavage for the removal of clotted blood can frequently be omitted. Two questions important for the further management can almost always be answered: (a) does the patient continue to bleed actively? and (b) does the bleeding come from the esophagus or from more distal areas? Besides the exact localization of the site of bleeding, other "potential" bleeding sites are frequently discovered that are not responsible for the acute hemorrhage. Emergency endoscopy requires a certain amount of endoscopic experience; it is particularly effective if a skilled team is available around the clock (see also p. 107).

2.1.6 Contraindications

There are only few absolute contraindications to an elective endoscopic examination. First is the uncooperative or undisciplined patient who will endanger not only himself but also the instrument. If cooperation is lacking, one should omit the examination. Acute corrosive or phlegmonous esophagitis is an absolute contraindication; particularly in cases of acute acid or lye burns, utmost caution is recommended. Caution is also necessary in cases of an aneurysm of the ascending aorta that may have led to a thinning of the esophageal wall.

Relative contraindications are pulsion diverticula, extreme kyphoscoliosis, large goiters, and large osteophytes of the cervical spine.

Esophageal varices are not a contraindication, even during acute hemorrhage. One need not be concerned about the possibility of causing bleeding by the endoscopic procedure.

2.1.7 Complications

The most dreaded complication is perforation. This can be largely avoided by carefully observing the contraindications. Whenever elastic resistance is encountered during introduction of the instrument or during its further advancement, the examination should be interrupted and the instrument pulled back to a point where clear vision can be obtained. Blind manipulation is extremely dangerous. Bleeding from biopsy sites occurs rarely. Tracheobronchial aspiration can, to a large degree, be prevented by positioning in the left lateral decubitus position. Adverse reactions to premedication and local anesthetics cannot be attributed to the procedure alone (see also p. 35).

References

1. Classen, M., Rösch, W., Frühmorgen, P., Seuberth, K., Demling, L.: Operative endoscopy: a diathermy hook for cutting of non-absorbable suture material. Endoscopy *6*, 42 (1974)
2. Frühmorgen, P., Jenny, S., Classen, M., Bäuerle, H., Koch, H.: Anamnese bei Ulcus und Narben im Bulbus duodeni. Dtsch. Med. Wochenschr. *97*, 188 (1972)
3. Ida, K., Kohli, Y., Shimamoto, K., Hashimoto, Y., Kawai, K.: Endoscopic findings of fundic and pyloric gland area using dye scattering method. Endoscopy *5*, 21 (1973)
4. Jenny, S., Frühmorgen, P., Classen, M., Bauerle, H., Demling, L.: Endoskopisch-radiologische Diagnostik des Bulbus duodeni. Dtsch. Med. Wochenschr. *97*, 118 (1972)
5. Pohl, W., Flachsenberg, E., Elster, K.: Endoscopic-bioptical diagnosis of antral mucosa within the duodenal stump. Endoscopy *4*, 162 (1972)
6. Rösch, W., Weidenhiller, S., Fuchs, H. F.: Endoskopie der Speiseröhre. Radiologe *13*, 361 (1973)
7. Stadelmann, O., Paul, F.: Endoskopische Diagnose der Oesophagusvarizen. Endoscopy *1*, 49 (1969)

2.2

Endoscopy of the Postoperative Stomach

B. C. MANEGOLD

Endoscopic inspection of gastric remnant and adjacent duodenal or jejunal segments reveals local postoperative abnormalities with a high degree of success. Surgical complications during the first postoperative days [12] and disturbances occurring years later can be recognized endoscopically when other diagnostic methods fail.

2.2.1 Instruments

For endoscopy of the postoperative stomach, a standard fiber endoscope with end-viewing optics, flushing and suctioning device, and flexibility of the tip in all directions is usually sufficient. With these instruments, the afferent and efferent loop of a Billroth II anastomosis can be intubated under direct vision, and surgically created narrowed (fundoplication) and widened areas (pyloroplasty) can be passed easily [1]. Retrograde duodenoscopy and cannulation of the papilla of Vater after the Billroth II partial gastrectomy are best attempted with an end-viewing instrument.

An anastomotic ulcer in the roof of an anastomosed jejunal loop can be better recognized with a slender, side-viewing duodenoscope. Narrow anastomoses and feeding gastrostomies can be passed with the small-caliber pediatric scopes.

The gastrocamera is not suitable for routine diagnostic evaluation of the postoperative stomach; it gives no information about the esophagus and the anastomosed intestinal loops.

A powerful suction apparatus is used to remove the frequently copious bile-stained intestinal secretions. If required, a defoaming agent is diluted with water and aimed through the biopsy channel under direct vision at the area covered with foam. Biopsy forceps with a central spike and long jaws are recommended because they yield larger tissue particles. These forceps, however, are not suitable for side-viewing instruments; in this situation, one must rely on the routine forceps. Biopsy specimens obtained with a diathermy snare will include the entire cross section of the mucosa to the muscularis mucosae, even in the presence of giant folds [11]. A special endoscopy table is not needed since special positioning of the patient is not necessary. An X-ray TV monitor will facilitate the location of the duodenal stump in a Billroth II stomach with a coexisting jejunojejunostomy.

2.2.2 Patient Preparation

In considering premedication, one has to consider that endoscopy of the postoperative stomach may take longer than usual and that it may be painful due to fixation of the gastric stump by adhesions. An analgesic is required if inspection of the duodenal stump is desired in the presence of a Billroth II anastomosis. Premedication is accomplished with atropine 0.5 mg intravenously and 10–20 mg of benzoctamine (Tacitin); if necessary, add 50–100 mg meperidine with levallorphan (Dolantin Spezial). Immediately thereafter and after pharyngeal anesthesia with lidocaine (Xylocain), the fiberscope, lubricated with mepivacaine gel (Scandicain), is introduced with the patient in the supine position. Secretions accumulating in the pharynx are removed by an aide using an additional suction apparatus independent of the gastroscope.

Knowledge of the X-ray findings and the surgical report are desirable but are not an absolute necessity. The endoscopist will have to define the surgically altered anatomy of the stomach and interpret it correctly by himself. For endoscopy of a recently operated stomach, however, the surgical details must be known so that this higher-risk examination can be performed as fast and as purposefully as possible.

2.2.3 Postprocedure Care

The postprocedure care follows the rules of general endoscopy [3,6]. Outpatients are unfit to drive and work on the day of the examination if they have received meperidine. They can go home by taxi after a rest period of 30–60 min without an escort. We ask them not to use public transportation. The patient is unfit to drive for 6 h if premedication was limited to atropine and benzoctamine (Tacitin).

2.2.4 Technique

During examination of a patient with previous gastric surgery, it should be remembered that considerable esophageal reflux of intestinal secretions can occur following anastomosis of the esophagus to the antrum or the jejunum. Suction must be constantly available during introduction of the instrument. A Billroth II stomach requires inspection of the gastrojejunostomy from the gastric as well as the jejunal side [10]. The suture line on the lesser curvature may be short or long, prominent in a pseudopolypoid fashion or recessed like a pseudodiverticulum. The opening of the anastomosis may be unusually wide or narrow. Its margin is either round and smooth or has a knobby appearance due to the folds radiating into it. Remnants of the surgical seromuscular suture [7] may be visible many years following the resection, particularly in the left or right commissure and mainly posteriorly. External injection of indigocarmine into abdominal wall fistulas will help identify fistulas originating from anastomoses or the duodenal stump. Endoscopic removal of sutures can result in healing of fistulas. The presence of a jejunojejunostomy indicates the presence of an antecolic gastroenterostomy [1].

For the assessment of a peptic ulcer of the jejunum, it is recommended to biopsy the ulcer margin to demonstrate its benign nature, to obtain a snare biopsy from the gastric remnant to exclude glandular hyperplasia of the mucosa, and to biopsy the duodenal stump to exclude a remnant of antral mucosa. Chromography with Congo red for the demonstration of antral remnants proximal to the anastomosis has not become common practice.

Retroflexion of the gastroscope is possible without difficulty in the resected stomach, even after re-resection. Incarceration of the instrument has been reported with the older types of fiberscopes. As a rule, retroflexion cannot be accomplished after esophagoantrostomy, or after subtotal distal resection, since the remaining gastric lumen matches only the diameter of the anastomosed jejunum. In cases of total gastrectomy with jejunal interposition according to Longmire, the esophagojejunostomy and jejunoduodenostomy may be inspected for dehiscence of suture lines and recurrence of carcinoma. The interposed loop is evaluated for the diameter of the lumen, color of the mucosa, and villous atrophy. Following selective proximal vagotomy, undisturbed peristalsis of the antrum, a circular pylorus, and absence of reflux of duodenal secretions proves that the operation was anatomically and functionally correct.

2.2.5 Indications

Early and late symptoms should be evaluated endoscopically in the postoperative stomach. The X-ray findings may thus be expanded in many ways [4]. Routine follow-up examinations at 6-month intervals following curative gastric resection for carcinoma are designed for early discovery of recurrences. Unfortunately, recurring cancer is more frequently present on the serosal side than in the mucosa. Endoscopic evaluation 10–20 years following partial gastrectomy for peptic ulcer disease is performed to detect a primary carcinoma in the gastric remnant that occurs with increased frequency as early as 7 years after the operation. Following endoscopic polypectomies, the patient remains under endoscopic surveillance until it has been demonstrated that the polypectomy was complete and that recurrence is unlikely. Nevertheless, a hyperplastiogenic polyp of the stomach may indicate an increased tendency of the mucosa for proliferation with an attendant risk of malignancy [2]. Therefore, follow-up examinations at 1–2 year intervals are indicated following polypectomy.

The completeness of a vagotomy can be checked by endoscopy [5,9]. Several weeks following vagotomy with pyloroplasty, a functional occlusion of the gastric outlet develops that can be demonstrated at endoscopy and prevents duodenogastric reflux [8]. The incidence of chronic atrophic gastritis following vagotomy for duodenal ulcer is still unknown. Also unknown is the frequency at which carcinoma develops from this atrophic mucosa. For this group of patients, no rational schedule for follow-up examinations has, so far, been established. Following vagotomy for a gastric ulcer, healing and scarring must be followed up very carefully to exclude a carcinoma, even if the ulcer was excised locally.

Bleeding in the operated stomach can be seen at endoscopy during the first postoperative hours from all lines of resection and anastomosis. If a deep duodenal ulcer was left behind during a Billroth II resection, this ulcer in the duodenal stump may bleed massively. Postoperative bleeding from erosions of the esophagus may be caused by introduction of a nasogastric tube during surgery.

Edema and hematomas at the anastomosis that cause postoperative gastric retention can be expressed toward the efferent loop by careful dilatation of the anastomosis with the tip of the instrument. Drainage of secretions can thereby be re-established and postoperative vomiting abolished. Routine endoscopic follow-up prior to discharge from the hospital of all patients undergoing gastric surgery is neither indicated nor practical.

2.2.6 Contraindications

For the skilled examiner, no contraindications exist to gastroscopy of the operated stomach. A Billroth II stomach may be examined as early as a few hours following resection without endangering the suture lines, if specific questions need urgent answers. Following proximal gastric resection with anastomosis to the esophagus, early passage by instruments of large caliber should be avoided.

2.2.7 Complications

The perforation of a correctly placed suture line during an early postoperative endoscopy need not be feared. This is only possible if an incomplete perforation already existed. Dehiscence of sutures may manifest itself at endoscopy by the presence of bare threads of seromuscular suture, or as an ulcer. These early ulcers in the suture line, not the obligatory marginal necroses of the line of resection, must be treated with caution. One should never remove sutures prior to complete wound healing.

The most serious result of endoscopy in the postoperative stomach is an incorrect diagnosis since this may rapidly lead to irreparable consequences.

References

1. Bartelheimer, H., Maurer, H. J., Schreiber, H. W.: Magenoperation und Magenoperierter. Berlin: De Gruyter 1969
2. Bötticher, R., Bünte, H., Hermanek, P., Rösch, W.: Magenpolypen, Prognose und Therapie. Dtsch. Med. Wochenschr. *100*, 167–170 (1975)
3. Brühl, W., Krentz, K.: Lehrbuch und Atlas der Gastroskopie. Stuttgart: Thieme 1969
4. Cotton, P. B., Rosenberg, M. T., Axon, A. T. R., Davis, M., Pierce, J. W., Price, A. B., Stevenson, G. W., Waldram, R.: Diagnostic yield of fibre-optic endoscopy in the operated stomach. Br. J. Surg. *60*, 629–632 (1973)
5. Demling, L.: Der kranke Magen. München: Urban & Schwarzenberg 1970
6. Demling, L., Ottenjann, R., Elster, K.: Endoskopie und Biopsie der Speiseröhre und des Magens. Stuttgart: Schattauer 1972
7. Gear, M. W. L., Dowling, B. L.: Suture-line ulcer after gastric surgery caused by non-absorbable suture materials. Br. J. Surg. *57*, 356–358 (1970)
8. Heymann, H., Helwing, E., Martens, H. L.: Die endoskopische Beurteilung der Pyloroplastik nach selektiver proximaler Vagotomie. Med. Klin. *63*, 1925–1930 (1968)
9. Kusakari, K., Nyhus, L. M., Gillison, E. W., Bombeck, C. T.: An en-

doscopic test for completeness of vagotomy. Arch. Surg. *105*, 386–391 (1972)

10. MANEGOLD, B. C.: Endoskopische Befunde im operierten Magen. Fortschr. Med. *91*, 1015–1017 (1973)
11. MANEGOLD, B. C.: Operative Endoskopie am oberen Verdauungstrakt. In: Fortschritte der gastroenterolog. Endoskopie. LINDNER, H. (Ed.). Vol. IV. Baden-Baden: Witzstrock 1973
12. REHNER, M., SOEHENDRA, N., STOLZENBACH, K.: Frühzeitige postoperative Endoskopie. Dtsch. Med. Wochenschr. *98*, 1319–1323 (1973)

2.3

Postbulbar Duodenoscopy and Endoscopic Retrograde Cholangiopancreatography (ERCP)

M. CLASSEN

2.3.1 Instruments

The purpose of the examination will determine the choice of the instrument. If the area of interest is the duodenal bulb or the descending portion of the duodenum (D1 and D2), end-viewing instruments are used, as for esophagogastroduodenoscopy (see Sect. 2.1.1). Inspection of the distal duodenum, as well as of the papilla of Vater, requires a special side-viewing instrument, as does cannulation of the papilla Vater. A new instrument with changeable optical axis combines the advantages of both instrument types (Fig. 1). For ERCP, an X-ray unit with a high-resolution intensifier is absolutely necessary for precise control of the filling of the pancreatic ductal system with contrast medium [1].

2.3.2 Patient Preparation

Preparation for duodenoscopy with or without ERCP does not differ from that for esophagogastroduodenoscopy (Sect. 2.1). Spraying of the pharnyx with a local anesthetic facilitates introduction of the instrument. Atropine is given to inhibit vagovagal reflexes, triflupromazine (Vesprin) as an antiemetic, meperidine (Demerol) as a sedative, hypnotic, and analgesic agent. Diazepam (Valium) in individual doses may be used in place of the latter two drugs. The premedication is designed to minimize the unpleasantness of the examination for the patient and to keep him cooperative at the same time. Since psychologic preparation is important, the entire course of the procedure should be described in a gentle and open manner.

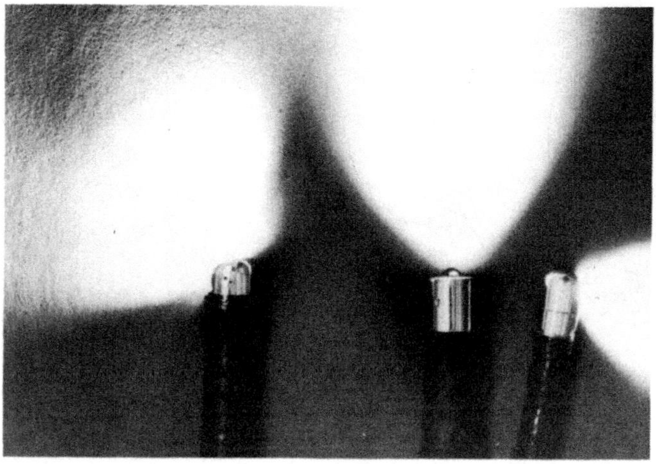

Fig. 1. Duodenoscopes with different optical systems: variable optics (PFS Machida; optical axis lateral—anterior); forward-viewing instrument (TX7, ACMI); side-viewing instrument (JF-B2, Olympus).

2.3.3 Postprocedure Care

Premedication and potential complications determine the follow-up observation of the patient. Endoscopists who examine their patients without premedication generally discharge them immediately following the procedure. Sedatives or tranquilizers, however, impair the patient's ability to react and his fitness to drive. One must make sure, therefore, that the patient is transported home by an escort following the examination. Symptoms of possible complications such as bleeding or perforation must be explained to the patient and the relatives.

We observe the patients in the hospital for 24 h following endoscopic biopsy procedures. Pulse and blood pressure are checked regularly and recorded. Following ERCP, we extend the follow-up observation period to 48 h because inflammatory complications in the pancreas may not manifest themselves until the 2nd day.

2.3.4 Technique

Introduction of end-viewing instruments into the duodenum rarely presents difficulties. The same is true for side-viewing instruments, although a few standard manipulations must be learned. Following inspection of the stomach, the instrument is placed directly in front of the pylorus (Fig. 2). The tip is then lifted upward so that the pylorus disappears from the field

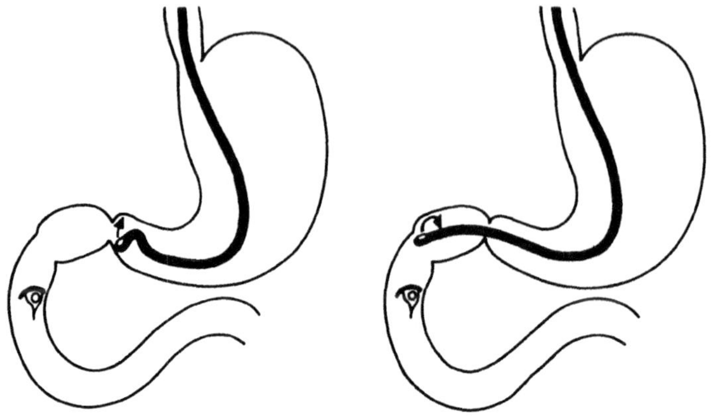

Fig. 2. Intragastric position of duodenoscope before and after passing the pylorus.

of vision and the lesser curvature comes into view. The instrument is advanced at this time and passes through the pylorus with a slight, palpable jerk. After insufflation of a small amount of air, one recognizes the duodenal bulb by the yellowish mucosa, which shows villi on close inspection. The optic is directed toward the superior portion, so that one has to rotate the instrument clockwise by 180° to look into the descending portion (D2). The instrument is now advanced further and the abovementioned 180° rotation reversed. By this maneuver, the papilla of Vater will appear in view. If inspection of more distal portions of the duodenum is indicated, the instrument is advanced further as necessary.

For ERCP, knowledge of the anatomy of the papilla of Vater and the lesser papilla, as well as their variants, is indispensable. The common bile duct and the main pancreatic duct can each enter with a separate papilla or jointly, in one papilla of Vater, with or without formation of a "common channel." Figure 3 (V. Becker) shows the important variants.

Before contrast material is injected into the papilla of Vater, one should make sure that catheter, adapter, and syringe contain no air bubbles that may interfere with the evaluation of radiographs. A wire functioning as a probe within the catheter is only rarely required when the opening is narrow. The angle at which the catheter is introduced into the papilla is of some importance. As as rule of thumb, the pancreatic duct is more likely to be filled if the catheter is introduced horizontally (Fig. 4) and the common bile duct more likely to be entered if the instrument is placed deeper, with the catheter tip pointing upward (Fig. 5). On the other hand, no infallible technique has yet been described for the selective visualization of the ductal system desired [5]. Occasionally, one has to turn the patient, who at the beginning of the examination is lying on his left side or on his

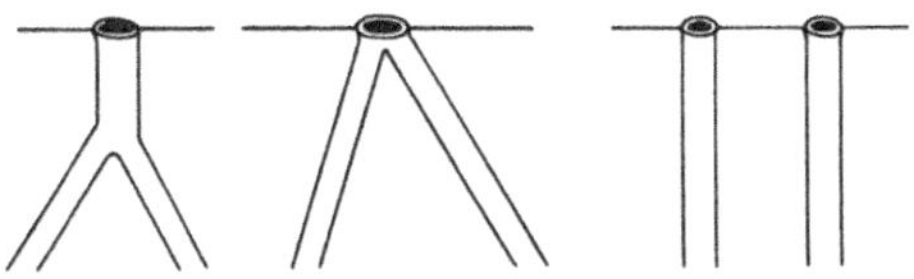

Fig. 3. The main variants of the entry of common bile and main pancreatic ducts into the duodenum (according to V. Becker).

abdomen, slowly onto his back; the catheter tip in the ampulla of Vater thus changes its position so that the common bile duct may be filled. With a good technique, pancreatography will be successful in more than 90% and cholangiography in over 85% of all patients.

For optimal radiographic imaging of the pancreatic and biliary duct system, the following approach is recommended:

1) Observe filling in the left lateral or prone position. Early films of the region of the papilla.
2) Films of the filled duct system/systems in the prone or supine position, possibly also in the right lateral decubitus position.
3) Fluoroscopy under rotation with spot films of individual segments.
4) Gradual compression, particularly if the biliary duct system is dilated.
5) Observation and timing of the drainage of the contrast material. The contrast material should have drained from both ductal systems within 10 min.

Removal of Tissue. The biopsy technique for tumors of the duodenum or the papilla of Vater with forceps or snare requires no special discussion. Additional cytology brushings under visual control will probably enhance the diagnostic yield. If a carcinoma of the pancreas or biliary tree is suspected, a catheter filled with normal saline can be advanced toward the

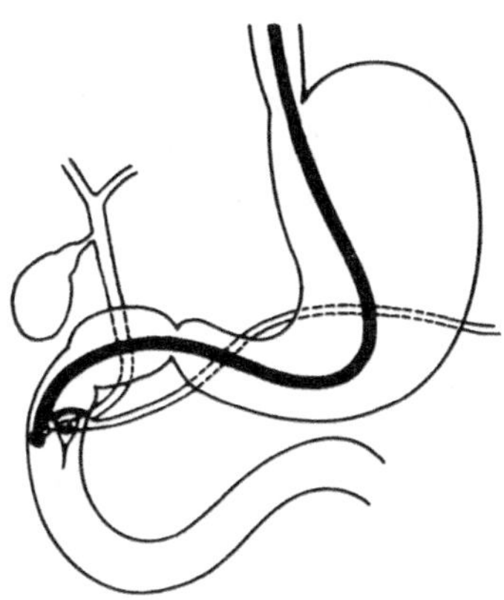

Fig. 4. Horizontal introduction of the catheter into the papilla favors intubation of the pancreatic duct.

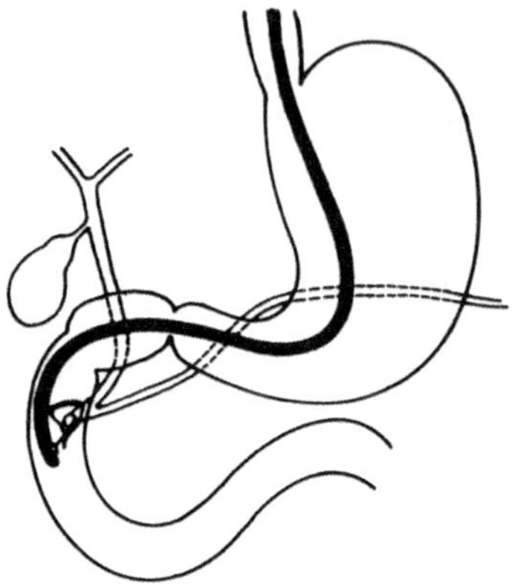

Fig. 5. Intubation aimed craniad for visualization of the common bile duct.

lesion after the contrast material has been drained from the ductal system and secretions originating in the suspicious area can be aspirated. Cytologic studies and carcinoembryonic antigen determination in the secretions obtained by selective aspiration will supplement suspicious ERCP findings. Miniaturized brushes that can be used to obtain tissue particles from the suspicious area under radiographic control are a further aid (see also Sect. 1.6).

2.3.5 Indications

Duodenoscopy is always indicated if clinical symptoms point toward localized changes in the upper small intestine. The most important symptoms are pain, bleeding, and obstruction. The latter manifests itself by vomiting. The vomitus is clear if the stenosis is proximal to the papilla and is bile-stained with infrapapillar obstruction. ERCP should be performed when clinical, laboratory, and radiographic findings indicate abnormalities of the papilla of Vater, the biliary tract, or the pancreas. In clinical practice, the most frequent indication is the cholestasis syndrome [6,8,9]. This is particularly true for patients in whom percutaneous transhepatic cholangiography (PTC) is not indicated (normal oral cholecystogram, postcholecystectomy syndrome, etc.) or contraindicated (e.g., sepsis, coagulopathy) [4].

2.3.6 Contraindications

The relative and absolute contraindications for duodenoscopy and ERCP are identical to those for the other endoscopic procedures (coagulopathy, cardiorespiratory decompensation). One must add viral hepatitis to this list because of possible contamination of the fiber endoscope by the viral agent. Since ERCP is not an aseptic technique and since spread of bacterial organisms may occur, control of acute inflammation in the area of examination (cholangitis, pancreatitis) should be attempted prior to the examination. If pancreatitis persists over a period of weeks, the study should be performed to diagnose and, possibly, correct the localized impairment of drainage that maintains the inflammation. Generally, however, we observe a safe interval of 6 weeks between the clinical and biochemical resolution of the inflammation and ERCP. Ultrasound examination of the upper abdomen prior to ERCP is recommended for the detection of pseudocysts of the pancreas (see below).

2.3.7 Complications

While intestinal injuries by the duodenoscope are theoretically possible, they are very rare. I am aware of only two (unpublished) cases of duodenal perforation. The papilla of Vater may bleed slightly after contact with the catheter, particularly if the catheter has been stiffened with a guide wire. Severe acute injuries of the papilla secondary to cannulation have not been reported. Occasionally, the tip of the catheter will be impaled in the epithelium of the ampulla, resulting in an intramural deposition of contrast material; because of its water solubility, however, it will disappear within a short time and will cause no complications. Following ERCP, inflammation of the organs studied occurs in 2%–3.5% of cases [1,7]. Cholangitis occurs particularly in the presence of stenoses or other obstructions to bile flow. Pancreatitis following pancreatography may occur even in the absence of organic obstruction. However, contrast material injection into pseudocysts is frequently followed by infection. The requirement for high-quality X-ray machines for this procedure is based on the high probability that injections of contrast material beyond the ductal system (parenchymography) will be followed by pancreatitis. A fatal outcome has been reported [7].

Prophylaxis and Countermeasures:

1) Careful observation of the filling of the pancreatic duct system with contrast material and avoidance of acinar filling.
2) Only minimal filling of pseudocysts.
3) Follow-up observation of the patient for 48 h. According to animal experiments and preliminary clinical experience, glucagon administration appears not to decrease the incidence of pancreatitis following ERCP.

References

1. Bilbao, M. K., Dotter, C. T., Lee, T. G., Katoni, R. M.: Complications of endoscopic retrograde cholangiopancreatography (ERCP). A study of 10.000 cases. Gastroenterology *70*, 314–320
2. Burwood, R. J., Davies, G. T., Lawrie, B. W., Blumgart, L. H., Salmon, P. R.: Endoscopic retrograde cholangiography—a review with a report of a collaborative series. Chir. Radiol. *24*, 397 (1973)
3. Classen, M., Hellwig, H., Rösch, W.: Anatomy of the pancreatic duct. A duodenoscopic-radiological study. Endoscopy *5*, 14 (1973)
4. Conn, H. D., Redeker, A. G., Zimmon, D. S.: PTC—ERC—An editor's dream. Gastroenterology *71*, 520 (1976)
5. Cotton, P.: Cannulation of the papilla of Vater by endoscopy and retrograde cholangiopancreatography. GUT 13, 1014 (1972)
6. Morrissey, J. F.: Cholangiography. N. Engl. J. Med. *289*, 266 (1973)
7. Ruppin, H., Ammon, R., Ettl, W., Classen, M., Demling, L.: Acute pancreatitis after endoscopic-radiological pancreaticography (ERP). Endoscopy *6*, 94 (1974)
8. Vennes, J. A., Jacobson, J. R., Silvis, S. E.: Endoscopic cholangiography for biliary system diagnosis. Ann. Intern. Med. *80*, 61 (1974)
9. Wurbs, D., Classen, M.: Bedeutung der endoscopisch retrograden Cholangio-Pankreatographie für die Differenzierung der Cholestase. Dtsch. Med. Wochenschr. *101*, 291–293 (1976)

2.4
Enteroscopy

H. KOCH

The esophagus, stomach, duodenum, colon, and cecum have become accessible to complete inspection by the development of modern fiberglass endoscopes. Enteroscopy, i.e., endoscopy of the jejunum and ileum, closes the last gap of gastrointestinal endoscopy.

Enteroscopy may be performed in several ways:

1) Attempt at total enteroscopy with the aid of a transintestinal guide
2) Partial enteroscopy
   a) Examination of the upper duodenum with the end-viewing endoscope as part of esophagogastroduodenoscopy
   b) Deep duodenoscopy with the side-viewing endoscope has as its primary goal the cannulation of the papilla of Vater; however, the intestinal lumen can be visualized as far as the ligament of Treitz and beyond
   c) Endoscopy of the upper jejunum with the enteroscope (without transintestinal guide)
   d) Retrograde endoscopy of the terminal ileum with the colonoscope
   e) Intraoperative enteroscopy

2.4.1 Instruments

So far, only Olympus prototypes have become available for total enteroscopy. These instruments are of the SIS-D type with a working length of 2 and 3 m and a diameter of 11 mm. Experience has shown that the 2-m endoscopes are sufficiently long for our technique of inspection of the

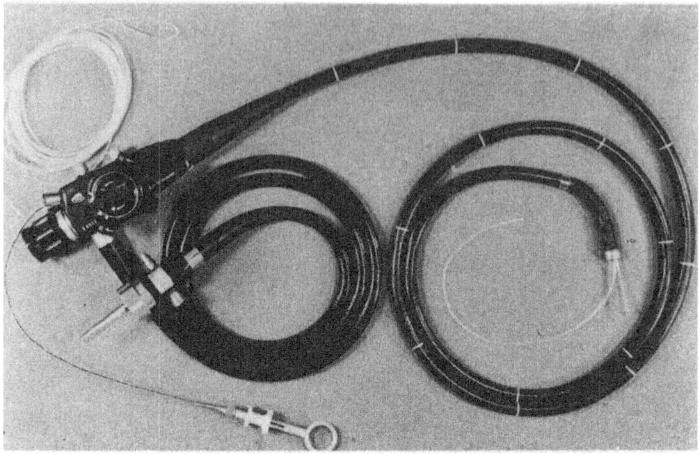

Fig. 1. Enteroscope, type SIS-D, Olympus Optical.

small intestine to the terminal ileum. They are available with one or two instrument channels. The tip of the instrument can be actively deflected by 150° upward, 120° downward, and by 90° to the right and the left. Lens flushing, aspiration of intestinal contents, and air insufflation are easily accomplished with the usual trumpet valves (Fig. 1).

The Olympus SIF-B endoscope (Fig. 2) is used for the examination

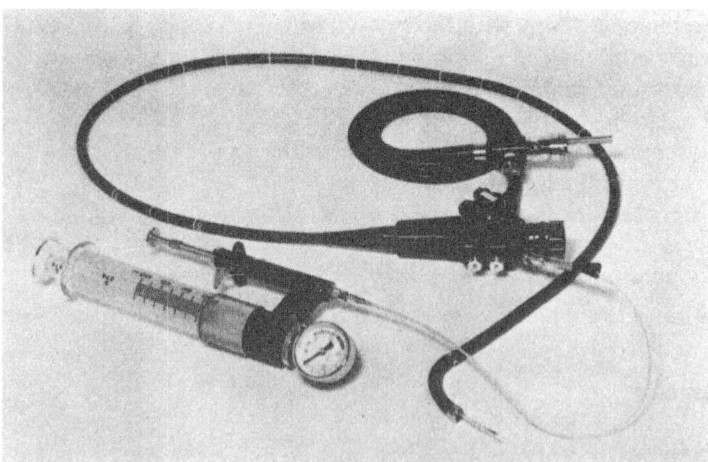

Fig. 2. Enteroscope, Olympus SIF-B.

of the upper jejunum without a transintestinal guide. This is an end-viewing instrument with a working length of 161 cm and an external diameter of 10 mm. Deflection of the tip and other technical data correspond to those of the above-mentioned enteroscope.

Another enteroscope provided by Olympus is being tested at the present time. This instrument corresponds in its outer diameter and in its design to the GIF-P2 endoscope with a working length of 175 cm, an external diameter of 9 mm, and an instrument channel 2 mm in diameter.

Like all other endoscopic examinations of the gastrointestinal tract, enteroscopy, with or without a transintestinal guide, is performed in patients who have fasted for at least 12 h. It is, however, advisable not to give any solid food for 24 h prior to the examination.

2.4.2 Patient Preparation

The premedication is similar to that used for esophagogastroduodenoscopy. One-half hour prior to the examination, while still on the ward, the patient receives 10–20 mg triflupromazine (Vesprin) and 0.5 mg atropine intramuscularly. Pharyngeal anesthesia is accomplished immediately prior to the examination with a 1% solution of a local anesthetic agent. In addition, 50–100 mg of meperidine with levallorphan (Dolantin Spezial) is given intravenously. During the examination, 20–40 mg butylscopolamine (Buscopan) can be given intramuscularly or intravenously, as necessary to relax the small bowel. Preparation customary for colonoscopy is required for retrograde endoscopy of the terminal ileum.

2.4.3 Postprocedure Care

Special postprocedure care after enteroscopy is generally not required. After removal of several biopsy specimens, however, it is recommended, as with all other endoscopic procedures, that the patient be observed for at least 5 h for possible bleeding.

2.4.4 Technique

A special technique had to be developed for total enteroscopy since the transfer of force to the tip of the instrument, necessary for the introduction of the instrument into the more distal segments of the small bowel, becomes a major problem. The pull-through procedure proved to be the most practical and successful method. A Teflon guide is passed throughout the in-

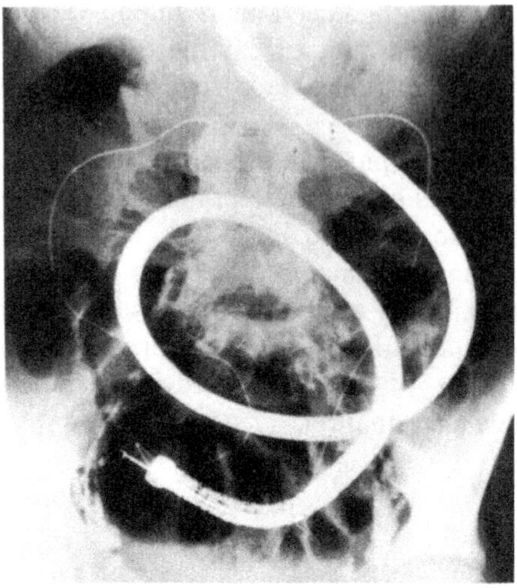

Fig. 3. Enteroscope: tip of the instrument with advanced biopsy forceps and transintestinal guide in the terminal ileum.

testine and is threaded through the instrument channel; with gradual pushing from above and pulling from the anus, the tip of the instrument can be kept in the axis of the intestinal lumen. If an enteroscope with only one instrument channel is used, no tissue biopsies can be obtained. Therefore, an endoscope with two instrument channels is preferable (Fig. 3).

A Teflon catheter, 1.8 mm in diameter, proved useful as an intestinal guide. A bag filled with buckshot is attached to its tip to facilitate passage. This Teflon catheter is first introduced through the nose and brought out again through the mouth. Then the bag with buckshot is attached and swallowed by the patient. After complete transintestinal passage (2–6 days), the guide can be filled with contrast material. It can then be detected radiographically, which simplifies introduction of the enteroscope considerably and allows one to ascertain its position in the small intestine.

The enteroscope can be advanced by this technique into the terminal ileum and, occasionally, into the proximal colon. The SIF-B instrument as well as the prototype of the GIF-P series can be advanced about 50 cm into the upper jejunum without the transintestinal guidc. The terminal ileum can be reached in about 80% of cases with one of the standard colonoscopes.

2.4.5 Indications

a) Diarrhea of undetermined origin
b) Clinically or radiographically suspected Crohn's disease
c) In established Crohn's disease, for exact endoscopic determination of extent of the disease

d) Clinical or radiographic suspicion of intestinal tumors
e) Intestinal bleeding of undetermined origin

2.4.6 Contraindications

Enteroscopy with a transintestinal guide and retrograde examination of the terminal ileum are contraindicated in the presence of acute inflammatory processes of the small and large intestine. No contraindications exist for oral enteroscopy without transintestinal guide.

2.4.7 Complications

Among 50 enteroscopies with transintestinal guide, one perforation of the terminal ileum occurred. This required immediate surgical intervention. The patient survived. Deyhle described multiple fissures of the small intestine after vigorous pulling on the transintestinal guide.

Complications of enteroscopy without transintestinal guide, as well as those of retrograde enteroscopy, correspond to those of esophagogastroduodenoscopy and colonoscopy.

2.4.8 Assessment

The diagnostic yield of enteroscopy with the use of a transintestinal guide is disappointing, with the exception of the evaluation of the extent of Crohn's disease.

The loops of small intestine are telescoped in harmonica fashion during introduction of the enteroscope. During withdrawal, therefore, when the intestine is actually examined, entire loops slide rapidly past the lens, preventing a definite assessment. In addition, enteroscopy with the transintestinal guide is frequently very painful to the patient and is associated with a high radiation exposure. For these reasons, this method has been almost completely abandoned.

At present, attempts are being made to perform enteroscopy without a transintestinal guide. Complete inspection of jejunum and ileum, however, is not possible. This limitation of the endoscopic evaluation of the small intestine is acceptable since most malignant tumors of the small intestine, particularly carcinomas and lymphomas, are located near the ligament of Treitz, most inflammatory processes are diffuse and can therefore be picked up by blind aspiration biopsy, and diagnostic evaluation of Crohn's disease is usually possible by retrograde inspection of the terminal ileum.

Enteroscopy with or without the use of a transintestinal guide has failed in the evaluation of occult gastrointestinal bleeding. Angiography is the method of choice in these patients.

2.4.9 Summary

These endoscopic procedures allow routine inspection of the duodenum, the upper portions of the jejunum, and the terminal ileum; thus, most malignant tumors of the small intestine can be recognized endoscopically, and the difficult differential diagnosis of Crohn's disease can be accomplished. Diffuse inflammatory diseases of the small bowel can be evaluated by blind aspiration biopsy. Enteroscopy has failed in the diagnostic evaluation of occult sources of bleeding in the small intestine.

References

1. CLASSEN, M., FRÜHMORGEN, P., KOCH, H., DEMLING, L.: Enteroskopie: Fiberendoskopie von Jejunum und Ileum. Dtsch. Med. Wochenschr. *11*, 409–411 (1972a)
2. CLASSEN, M., FRÜHMORGEN, P., KOCH, H., DEMLING, L.: Peroral enteroscopy of the small and the large intestine. Endoscopy *4*, 157–160 (1972b).
3. KOCH, H.: Endoskopische Dünndarmdiagnostik. Symposium: Der kranke Dünndarm, Hamburg 1977
4. MORSON, B. C.: Histopathology of Crohn's Disease. Scand. J. Gastroenterol. *6*, 573 (1971)
5. SHINYA, H.: Total gastrointestinal endoscopy. Paper presented at the Annual Conf. Am. Soc. Gastroint. Endoscopy, New York 1973

2.5
Colonoscopy

P. FRÜHMORGEN

Endoscopic examination of the colon allows targeted morphologic and preoperative diagnostic evaluation of the entire colon and the adjacent terminal ileum [1–12].

2.5.1 Instruments

Truly flexible fiberglass endoscopes (Figs. 1 and 2) with variable operating length and different optical and mechanical properties are available. Short endoscopes are used for sigmoidoscopy and partial colonoscopy, long endo-

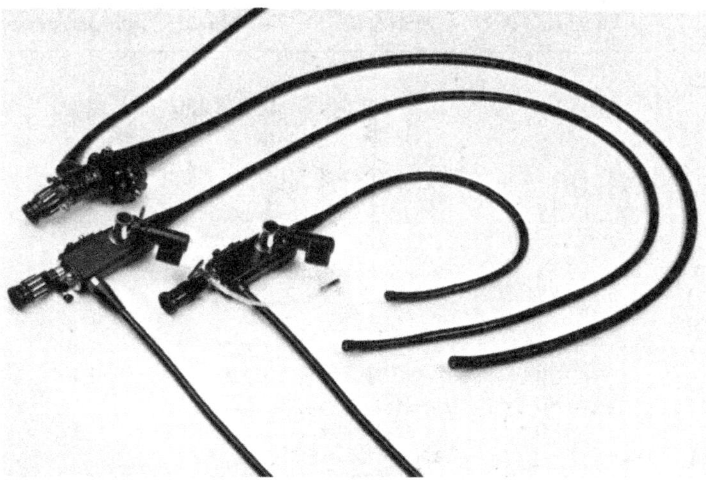

Fig. 1. Long colonoscope with two channels, type TX-92; colonoscope with one channel, type FX-91; and fiber sigmoidoscope, type F-91S (ACMI).

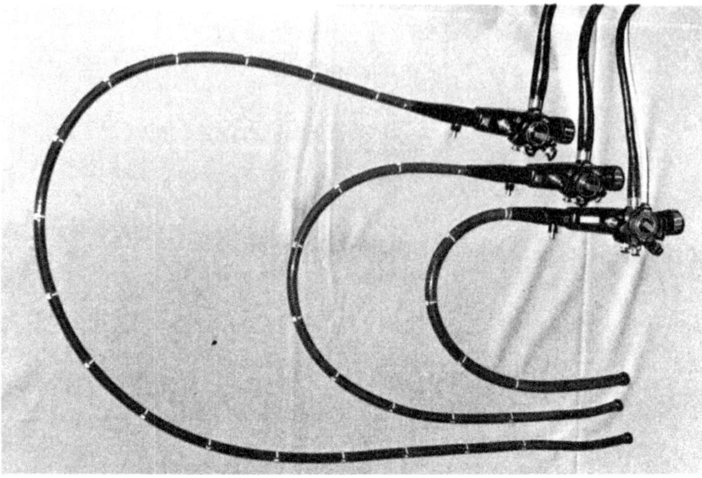

Fig. 2. Long colonoscope, type CF/LB3; short colonoscope, type CF/MB3; and fiber sigmoidoscope, type TCF-1S (Olympus).

scopes for high colonoscopy and ileoscopy by the anal route (manufacturers: ACMI, Olympus, Machida, Wolf). Table 1 summarizes the technical data of these instruments with end-viewing optics. All have an

Table 1. Technical data of colonoscopes.

Technical data	*ACMI F9-S/F9-L TX91R/TX91*	*Olympus CF-MB3/ LB3/IB*	*Machida FCS-M1/ FCS*	*Wolf sigmoidoscope*
Working length (mm)	1050/1650	1035/1785/ 1435	1050/1850	860
Diameter, rigid portion of tip (mm)	15	13.5	14.5	15.5
Length of the rigid portion of the tip (mm)	55	78	20.0	25.0
Deflection of tip				
Upward	180°	130°	120°	140°
Downward	180°	130°	120°	140°
To the right	180°	160°	120°	0
To the left	180°	160°	120°	0
Depth of visual field (mm)	10–200	10–100	7–45	5–∞
Angle of vision	75°	85°	60°	70°
Variable focus	0	0	0	+

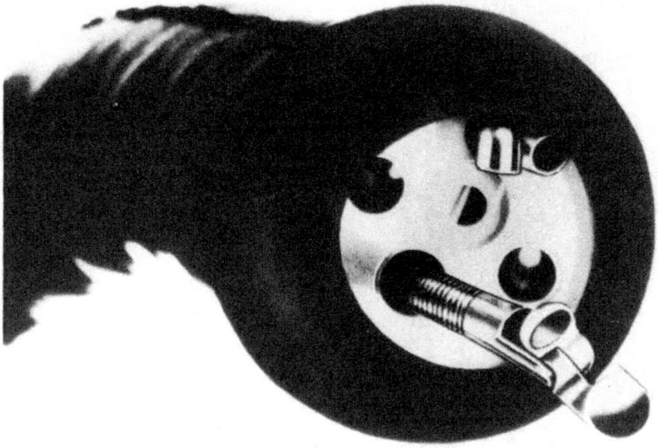

Fig. 3. End-viewing optics of a fiber colonoscope with various functional elements (instrument channel, light and image bundle, suction, flushing and insufflation device).

automatic or semiautomatic suction and flushing device, air insufflation, and an instrument channel (Fig. 3). The instrument tip of the colonoscopes in most frequent use can be flexed in four directions (Fig. 4) (Olympus, Machida) or can be flexed without interruption in any desired direction up to 180° with a single lever (ACMI).

Accessory instruments, such as biopsy forceps, retractable nylon brushes for cytologic studies, graduated measuring probes, and Teflon catheters for cannulation of fistula tracts and instillation of contrast material should be available. For documentation by film and photography, high quality 35-mm photographic and movie cameras (Super 8, 16 mm) with the appropriate adapter for connection with the ocular portion of the endoscope are necessary.

Partial stiffening of the colonoscope after successful straightening of the sigmoid is possible either with a Teflon-coated steel wire introduced through the instrument channel or with a plastic tube that can be introduced over the instrument. Using endoscopes of the last generation these measures are unnecessary. For therapeutic colonoscopy, particularly for excision of polypoid lesions, a high-frequency electrosurgery unit, high-frequency diathermy snares of varying size, grasping forceps, and a flexible coagulation electrode must be available (p. 111). An X-ray unit with image intensifier and TV monitor (Arcoskop 100-3D, Siemens) has proved useful to occasionally check the position of the instrument tip and findings, to straighten loops without risk, and to take single exposures for documentation.

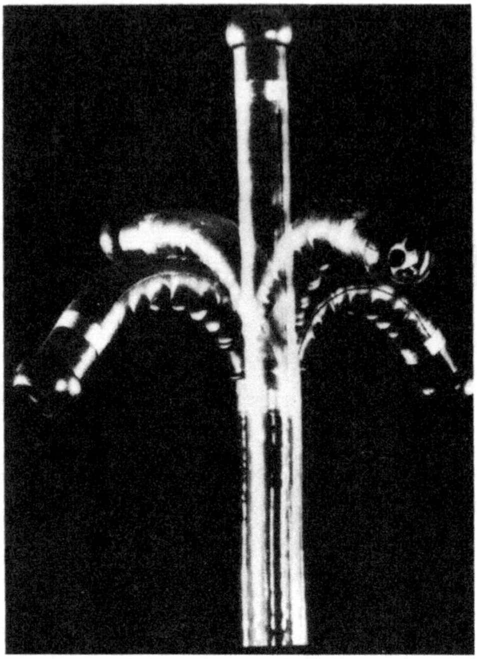

Fig. 4. Flexibility of the instrument tip in four directions up to 180° (Olympus).

2.5.2 Patient Preparation

Elective high colonoscopy requires patient selection. In comparison with radiographic examination of the colon, the endoscopic examination can be time-consuming and not without risk in less skilled hands. Less demanding preliminary examinations should be used to select for colonoscopy only those patients in whom a diagnosis cannot be made by simpler diagnostic procedures. As a rule, colonoscopy should be preceded by a detailed history and proctosigmoidoscopy. A technically unsatisfactory radiographic study of the colon is not an indication for colonoscopy. For biopsies and, in particular, polypectomies, the coagulation profile (prothrombin time, partial thromboplastin time, platelet count) and blood group should be determined.

Adequate cleansing of the colon is a requirement for successful colonoscopy. In addition to a liquid diet, we prescribe on the day preceding the procedure 125 cc of magnesium sulfate in the morning and afternoon and administer two high warm tap water enemas without addition of glycerol (clouding of the lens). Sigmoidoscopy alone requires only a cleansing enema and one administration of magnesium sulfate on the evening preceding the examination. Once the technique has been mastered, no premedication is required; however, one should discuss the need for the examination and its course with the patient.

2.5.3 Postprocedure Care

After an uneventful examination, intensive observation of the patient is not required. Only after polypectomies and other therapeutic interventions are patients kept in the hospital overnight so that possible delayed bleeding and perforations can be recognized and treated early.

2.5.4 Technique

After the colonoscope has been checked and found to be ready for use, the instrument tip and the distal end of the endoscope are lubricated with olive oil, better silicon oil. The anal canal is entered without the help of a speculum, with the patient in the left lateral decubitus position. The instrument should be advanced further only after the lumen of the rectal ampulla has been visualized by slight withdrawal of the instrument and concomitant air insufflation. Blind advancement of the colonoscope within the intraperitoneal sigmoid and colon will lead to formation of additional loops, which may be difficult or impossible to overcome. Any such attempt risks perforation. Only when the mucosa slides by the lens without difficulty and without developing pallor as the instrument is gingerly advanced is it safe to deviate from the requirement that the instrument always be introduced with the lumen in sight. If this manipulation remains unsuccessful, the instrument must be immediately withdrawn for a few centimeters; a second attempt can be made to pass the obstacle, or the position of the patient can be changed.

Complaints of discomfort by a patient who has not been premedicated are a valuable hint for the examiner to change his technique. The alternating insufflation and removal of air avoids overdistention of the colon and discomfort to the patient caused by this artificial meteorism.

The mucosa is examined in detail on the way out, after the colonoscope has been completely introduced and the instrument, and with it the intestinal loops, has been straightened; on the way in, the mucosa is only examined for purposes of orientation. Without straightening of the sigmoid it is impossible, as a rule, to examine the entire mucosal surface and to exclude the presence of lesions with confidence.

The intraperitoneal location of the sigmoid and its fixation to the mesocolon will lead to variable loop formations. Most of the loops, however, are the result of insufficient techniques and/or colonoscopes of former times with bad mechanical properties. These, however, can be reduced to certain basic configurations; their knowledge will facilitate the straightening maneuvers required for further introduction. For better communication, we refer to these loops according to their configurations as alpha, beta, phi, eta, and sigma forms (Fig. 5).

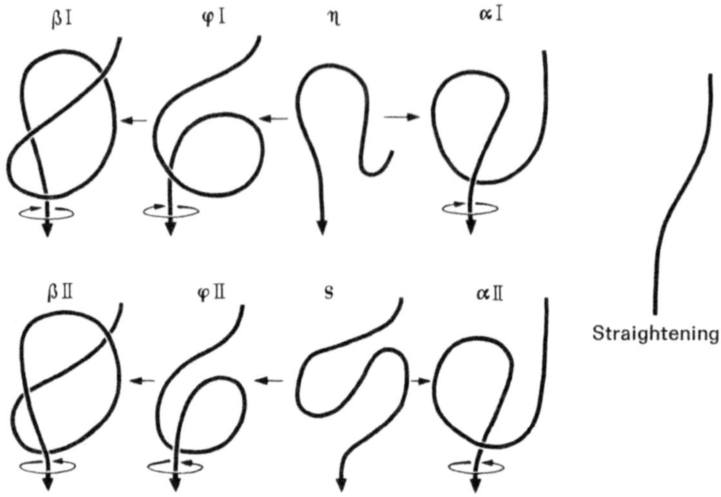

Fig. 5. Sigma loops (basic forms); straightening.

The goal of the first phase of introduction is the splenic flexure. It can be reached in most cases, without prior straightening, particularly in the presence of the common alpha configuration of the sigmoid (Fig. 6). Subsequently, the tip of the instrument is angled beyond the splenic flexure toward the transverse colon and is thereby fixed. The sigmoid loops can be straightened by pulling and rotating the distal end of the colonoscope (Fig. 6). The direction of rotation depends upon the relative arrangement of the superimposed sigmoid loops. If the crossing distal portion of the colonoscope is located anteriorly, the instrument is rotated toward the left; if it lies posteriorly, it is rotated clockwise, i.e., toward the right (Fig. 5, α I and II).

The rarer phi-shaped configuration of the sigmoid is the mirror image of the previously described alpha loop, and the manipulations required are analogous to those outlined for the straightening of the alpha configuration.

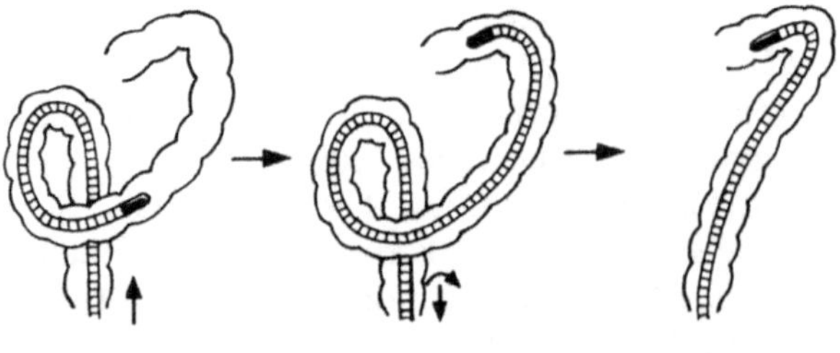

Fig. 6. Straightening of the sigmoid (alpha configuration).

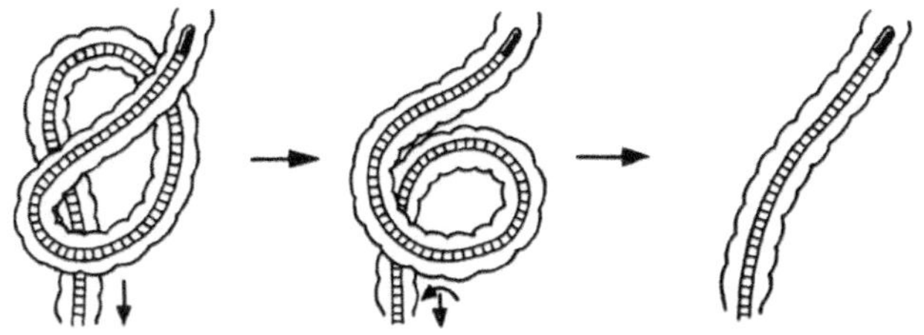

Fig. 7. Straightening of the sigmoid (beta configuration).

Further advancement of the instrument in the presence of a phi configuration without corresponding advancement of the instrument tip will result in a secondary beta configuration of the sigmoid (Fig. 5). It can easily be seen that this loop can again be reduced to a phi form simply by pulling at the colonoscope; thereafter, the instrument is completely straightened using the technique described for these configurations (Fig. 7).

The basic forms of all sigmoid loops, from which all other sigmoid configurations may develop by physiologic rotation, correspond to an eta or sigma configuration (Fig. 5). The sigma form, which gives this segment of intestine its name, is extremely rare. This configuration can only be passed after it has been transformed into an alpha loop by rotation (Fig. 5).

A common characteristic of both forms is that in some cases the colonoscope can initially only be advanced up to the transition of the sigmoid to the descending colon. Further advance of the instrument will only extend the sigmoid loop craniad without transfer of force to the instrument tip sufficient for its passage into the descending colon (Fig. 8).

The hand of an assistant pushing into the abdomen may anchor the medial aspect of the sigmoid loop in the pelvis and, thereby, facilitate further advancement in a given case. If not, one should attempt to straighten the sigmoid by fixing the tip of the instrument at the transition to the descending colon and simply pulling at the distal end of the colonoscope.

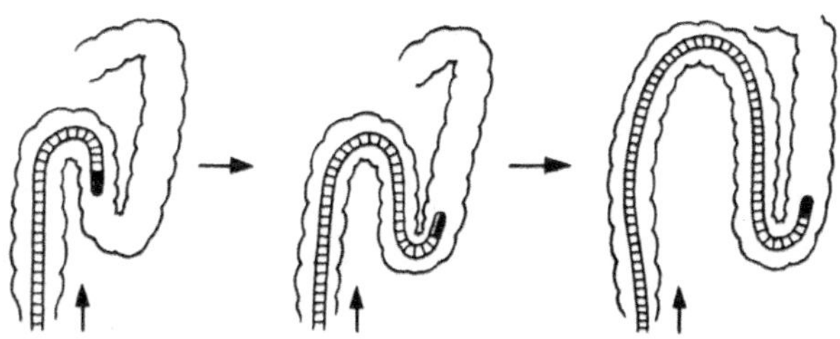

Fig. 8. Impossible passage of the sigmoid (eta configuration).

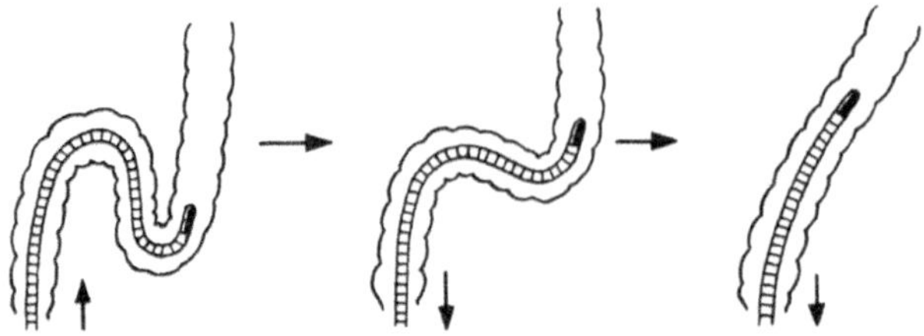

Fig. 9. Straightening of the sigmoid (eta configuration). First option.

If this manipulation is successful, the instrument tip will advance into the descending colon while the sigmoid is straightened (Fig. 9).

Another way to successfully pass the sigmoid is to transform an eta-shaped configuration into a more easily passable alpha loop by rotating the instrument counterclockwise 180° after the upper loop of the sigmoid has been reached. Thereafter, the tip of the instrument can be advanced to the splenic flexure; subsequently the sigmoid is straightened in the manner described (Fig. 10).

If the cecum is to be reached easily with the colonoscope in every case, straightening of the sigmoid and subsequent partial stiffening of the colonoscope are necessary. Stiffening, however, is not necessary with the newer generation of colonoscopes. To prevent formation of secondary loops and to facilitate sufficient transfer of force to the instrument tip, the colonoscope can be stiffened from outside by the hand of an assistant pushing into the abdomen or, if necessary, by introduction of a stiffening probe through the instrument channel or with the aid of a plastic tube, which is advanced over the instrument up to the handle prior to introduction of the colonoscope (Fig. 11).

The stiffening device should be advanced to about 10 cm distal to the splenic flexure. If a plastic tube is used, one must make sure that it is advanced only after the sigmoid has been completely straightened; otherwise, new loops will form or the intestinal wall may be injured (Fig. 12).

Passage of the transverse and descending colon constitutes the second

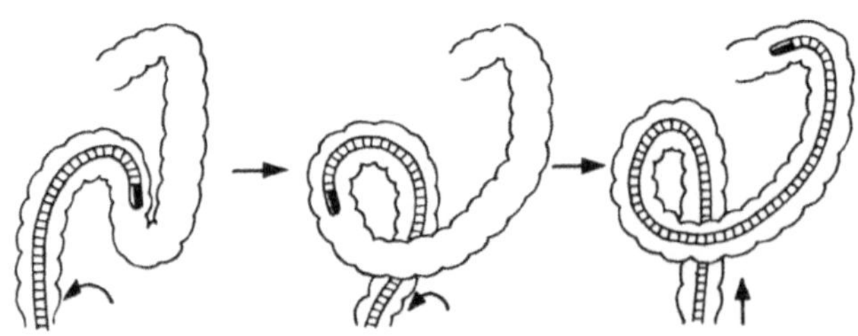

Fig. 10. Straightening of the sigmoid (eta configuration). Second option.

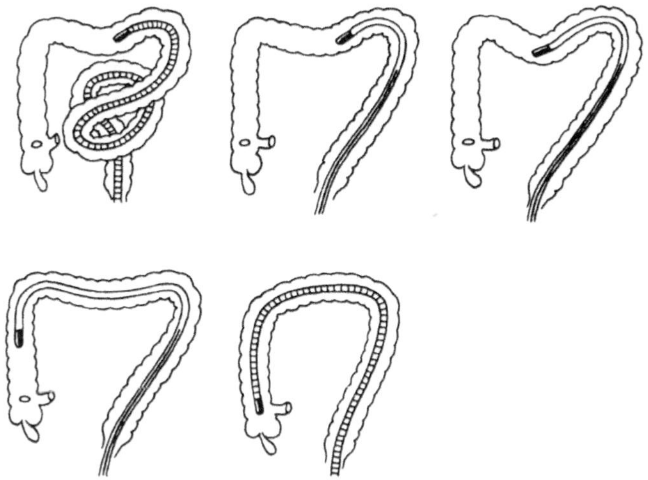

Fig. 11. Technique of introduction with stiffening device (plastic tube, Teflon-coated steel wire).

phase of high colonoscopy. Once the sigmoid has been negotiated and straightened, the most difficult part of the colonoscopy is over. A transverse colon with a deep downward arc or with an undulating course can, however, make further advancement difficult. Passage of such a transverse colon can be made easier if one can prevent it from sliding further downward by gradual external pressure (manually exerted by an assistant) (Fig. 14).

To lessen the pain of introducing the instrument into the ascending colon, the instrument tip should be fixed after the hepatic flexure is reached and the transverse colon straightened (Fig. 13). During this manipulation, however, the tip of the instrument may slip back into the midtransverse colon. This can be prevented by keeping the transverse colon straight by

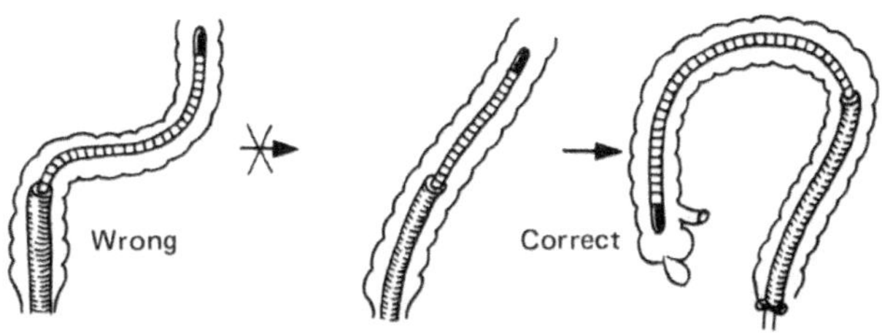

Fig. 12. Wrong and correct application of a plastic tube for partial stiffening of the colonoscope.

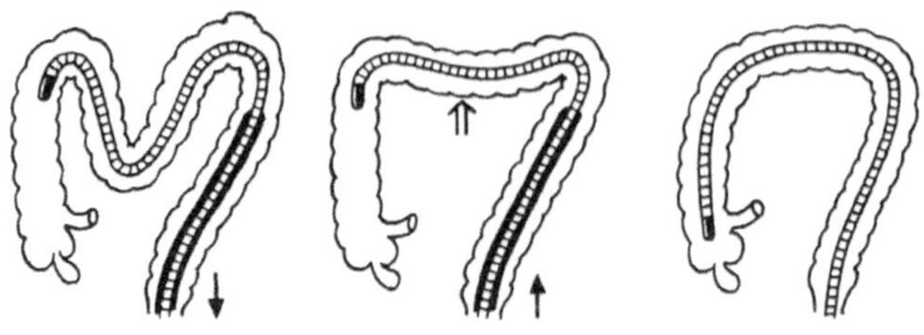

Fig. 13. Passage of a transverse colon with downward displacement after straightening and external fixation of the colonoscope.

external compression and by tilting the instrument tip into the ascending colon.

After these manipulations have been accomplished, the cecum can be reached in every instance and the terminal ileum in over 80% of cases. In view of the multitude of possible configurations of the colon and the variable techniques required by them, universally applicable rules and guidelines cannot be given.

2.5.5 Indications

Indications are based on history, clinical findings, and the results of the previously mentioned preliminary examinations (p. 90). Questionable or unclear X-ray findings, negative X-ray examinations in the presence of persistent abdominal complaints (diarrhea, constipation, discharge of blood, mucus and pus, tenesmus, incomplete obstruction), follow-up examination after surgical resection of malignant tumors of the colon, and established diseases with an increased risk for carcinoma are considered absolute indications. Preoperative histologic confirmation of the diagnosis and assess-

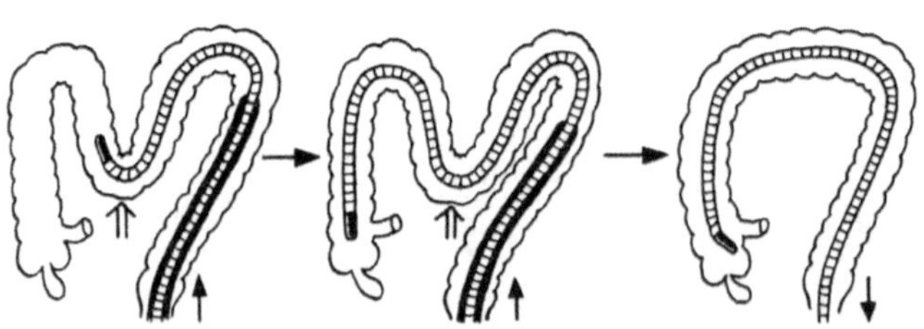

Fig. 14. Straightening of a transverse colon with U-shaped configuration.

ment of the severity and extent of pathologic processes help in the planning of surgery or may render it unnecessary.

Polypoid lesions are removed primarily for diagnostic purposes. The aim is an exact diagnosis and to avoid a surgical intervention that will put the patient at greater risk. Bleeding per rectum should be evaluated by colonoscopy only after a source of bleeding in the proximal gastrointestinal tract (p. 107) has been excluded by endoscopy. Follow-up of benign disorders and assessment of therapeutic results are relative indications [5,7].

2.5.6 Contraindications

To avoid complications, that is, perforation and increased bleeding, highly active inflammatory diseases of the colon, toxic megacolon, and peritonitis represent absolute contraindications.

Diverticulosis, as well as previous abdominal surgery, may make colonoscopy more difficult; however, they are not contraindications. The less experienced examiner should forego colonoscopy in these patients in view of the increased risk of complications.

2.5.7 Complications

In the hands of the experienced endoscopist, colonoscopy is an extremely low-risk procedure. Lack of skill or disregard for contraindications, however, can lead to perforation and bleeding, particularly in the hands of inexperienced examiners (Table 2).

Besides polypectomy, blind advancing of the colonoscope and biopsy of diverticula constitute the greatest risk for perforation of the colon. Free air on an upright film of the abdomen confirms the suspicion.

Minimal bleeding, such as contact bleeding in the presence of inflamed mucosa or after forceps biopsy, is harmless and will, as a rule, stop spon-

Table 2. Complications of colonoscopy.

Complications	*Severe bleeding*	*Perforations*	*Mortality*
Colonoscopies			
A/S/G/E, 1974: 25,298	12 (0.05%)	55 (0.22%)	2 (0.008%)
Erlangen, 1977: 3,432[a]	0	2(0.06%)	0
Frühmorgen, 1978: 35,892[a] (Survey, W. Germany)	3 (0.008%)	51 (0.14%)	7 (0.02%)

[a] Without polypectomies.

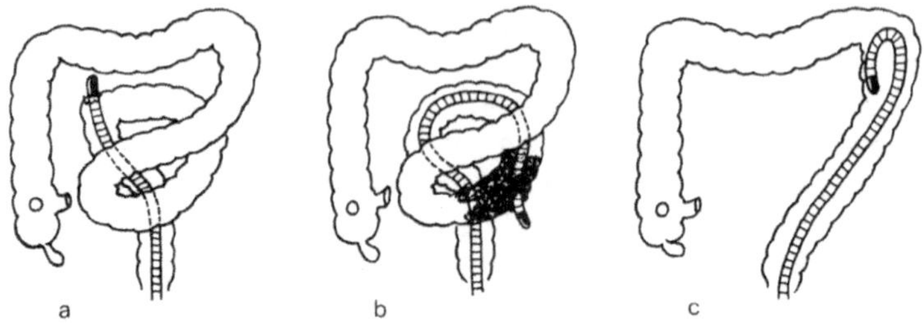

Fig. 15a–c. Possible complications due to inappropriate technique.

taneously. Biopsy of hemangiomas or colonic varices and mechanical removal of larger polypoid lesions by forceps may, however, lead to major hemorrhages.

Localized sources of bleeding should first be compressed with the biopsy forceps and observed while the instrument remains in place. If this approach is unsuccessful, one can attempt to achieve hemostasis by cautious electrocoagulation with a ballpoint electrode, or by laser coagulation. The application of vasoconstrictive agents to the site of bleeding is usually not successful since they will be washed off by the emerging blood.

In a normal colon, as well as in the presence of stenoses, lack of experience or careless introduction may lead to a harmless inversion of the instrument but also to avoidable perforations (Fig. 15). Even the use of an instrument as harmless as the biopsy forceps should be deliberate and under full view of the lumen. Bleeding, perforation of diverticula, as well as perforations of a thinned bowel wall could ensue (Fig. 16).

The examiner should not forget that blind areas may develop behind flexures and prominent haustra, even after optimal straightening. These require particularly careful maneuvering so that even the smallest lesions are not overlooked in these areas (Fig. 17).

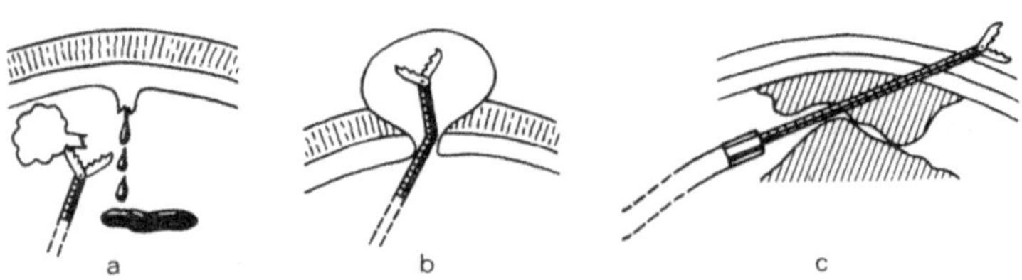

Fig. 16a–c. Complications due to abuse of biopsy forceps.

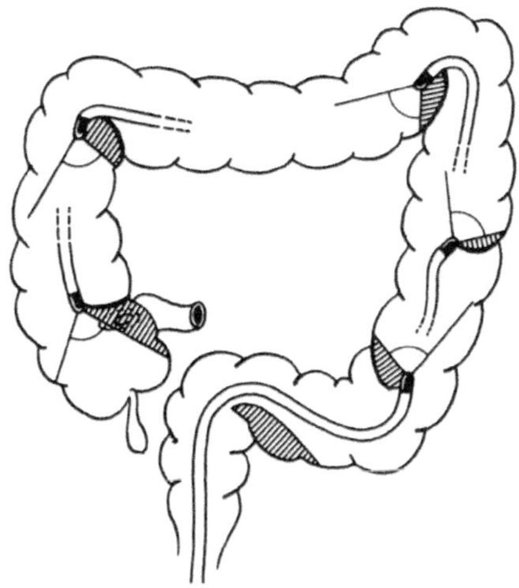

Fig. 17. Poorly visible or nonvisible areas with use of end-viewing optics.

References

1. Beck, K., Dischler, W., Helms, M. Oehlert, W.: Farbatlas der Endoskopie und Biopsie des Darmes. Stuttgart: Schattauer 1973
2. Demling, L., Classen, M., Frühmorgen, P.: Atlas der Enteroskopie. Springer Verlag, Heidelberg 1974. Berlin, Heidelberg, New York: Springer 1974
3. Deyhle, P.: A plastic tube for the maintenance of the straightening of the sigmoid colon during coloscopy. Endoscopy *4*, 224 (1972)
4. Deyhle, P., Demling, L.: Coloscopy—Technique, results, indications. Endoscopy *3*, 143 (1971)
5. Frühmorgen, P., Demling, L.: Complications of diagnostic and therapeutic colonoscopy in the Federal Republic of Germany. Endoscopy *2*, 146 (1979)
6. Frühmorgen, P.: Coloskopie—Vorbereitung, Technik, Ergebnisse. Fortschr. Med. *5*, 190 (1974)
7. Frühmorgen, P., Zeus, J., Classen, M.: Klinische Wertigkeit der Coloskopie. In: Fortschritte der gastroenterologischen Endoskopie. Lindner, H. (Ed.), vol. IV, S. Baden-Baden: Witzstrock 1973
8. Nagasako, K., Takemoto, T.: Endoscopy ot the ileocecal area. Gastroenterology *65*, 403 (1973)
9. Nagasako, K., Yazawa, C., Takemoto, T.: Observation of the terminal ileum. Endoscopy *1*, 45 (1971)
10. Nagy, G. S.: Fibrecolonoscopy. Med. J. Aust. *1*, 378 (1973)
11. Sakat, Y.: The technic of colonofiberscopy. Dis. Colon Rectum *15* (6), 403 (1972)
12. Williams, Chr., Muto, T.: Examination of the whole colon with the fibreoptic colonoscope. Br. Med. J. *3*, 278 (1972)

2.6

Protosigmoidoscopy and Proctoscopy

K. ARNOLD

The combination of these endoscopic procedures permits inspection of the anal canal, rectum, and varying portions of the sigmoid with rigid instruments up to 30 cm in length.

Careful digital examination of the anal canal and the distal portion of the rectal ampulla should be followed by proctosigmoidoscopy (PS). Proctoscopy, also termed anoscopy, is best performed as the final part of the examination.

2.6.1 Proctosigmoidoscopy

2.6.1.1 Instruments

All modern instruments use cold illumination. The time has passed for the small electric bulb to serve as light source.

Proctosigmoidoscopes with *distal* illumination (e.g., Wolf, Knittlingen, W. Germany) offer the highest light density since the glass fiber bundles end at the distal aperture. The ring of illumination, however, frequently becomes soiled by rectal contents. The instruments consist of one piece.

With instruments featuring *proximal* illumination (e.g., Storz, Tuttlingen, W. Germany), some light energy is lost during transmision through the tubular section. The light source, located in a detachable proximal part, is less likely to become obscured by feces and is easy to clean. This type of proctosigmoidoscope consists of two components: the expensive head piece that can be fitted with any number of inexpensive tubes of different diameters and lengths. Instruments of this type have found wide acceptance in clinics performing large numbers of examinations.

Disposable plastic instruments are satisfactory only when lateral loss of illumination is minimized by internal coating. They currently are relatively expensive and are suitable only when few examinations are performed and when the inconvenience of instrument cleaning needs to be considered.

2.6.1.2 Patient Preparation

PS can easily be carried out in ambulatory patients. Fasting and constipating medications are unnecessary. Preparation of the patient with laxatives is illogical since the examiner will then encounter a stream of liquid stool with continuous moistening of the mucosa under inspection. Multiple enemas are indicated only when there is reason to expect the mucosa to be covered by adherent material, such as after a barium enema examination. Hypertonic enemas cause mucosal secretion and hyperemia and wash out residual blood that may give a clue to a more proximal bleeding site. No special preparation is needed in most instances; defecation shortly before the procedure is sufficient for adequate visualization of the lumen within reach of the instrument.

When necessary, we administer an enema (olive oil or saline) 15 min prior to the examination. The patient preferably walks about and is examined immediately after he has evacuated his rectum.

2.6.1.3 Postprocedure Care

In routine cases, postprocedure care is not needed. For exceptions see Sect. 2.6.1.7.

2.6.1.4 Technique

The knee-elbow position on a flat surface has largely been abandoned in favor of adjustable examining tables. With these the kneeling patient is titled head-down and supports his weight with thighs, head, and arms (Fig. 1). Although this position tends to force the thighs into adduction, making the inspection of the anal region more difficult, the sigmoid colon unfolds and is easier to enter. Older individuals and patients with circulatory disorders cannot tolerate this position very long.

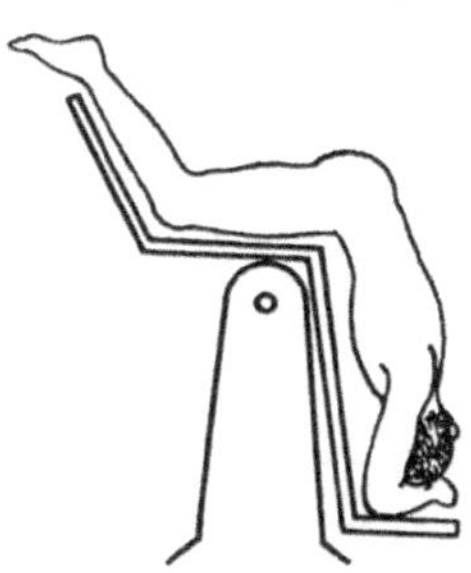

Fig. 1. Patient on the tilt table. The body weight is supported by the arms; the head is pushed laterally. The thigh muscles contract to apply counterpressure. Older patients can tolerate this head-down position only for short periods.

The lithotomy (supine) position appears more comfortable to the patient. It is less advantageous to the examiner, however, since the sigmoid descends into the true pelvis unless it is possible to tilt the bed or examining table slightly head-down.

We prefer the Sims's position. The patient lies on his left side with knees flexed and a sand bag under the left high (Fig. 2). The perianal region can be inspected easily, the patient is relaxed, and any wide surface may be used as an examining table.

When the digital examination, which should precede every PS, reveals a painful lesion in the anal canal (commonly an anal fissure), then the surrounding area should be infiltrated with 2–4 ml of a local anesthetic, using a thin needle. This will assure a relaxed patient and a painless examination. We perform PS under general anesthesia only on about 1 of 1500 occasions, mainly in the presence of stenoses of the rectum or at the rectosigmoid junction.

Our routine proctosigmoidoscope is 30 cm long and 16 mm in diameter, formerly considered a pediatric instrument. Its total diameter is 4 mm less than that of the usual adult proctosigmoidoscope. This facilitates deep introduction of the instrument tube because the rectosigmoid angulation is easier to negotiate and because the sigmoid lumen frequently is narrowed by diverticular disease in older patients. Children, by contrast, can easily be examined with wider instruments since their tissues are very elastic. The caliber of children's bowel movements confirms this impression.

The instrument is introduced blindly to the level and in the direction of the preceding digital exploration. Further advances are made under direct vision. The instrument should be withdrawn slightly when difficulties are encountered. The direction of the lumen is better recognized from the

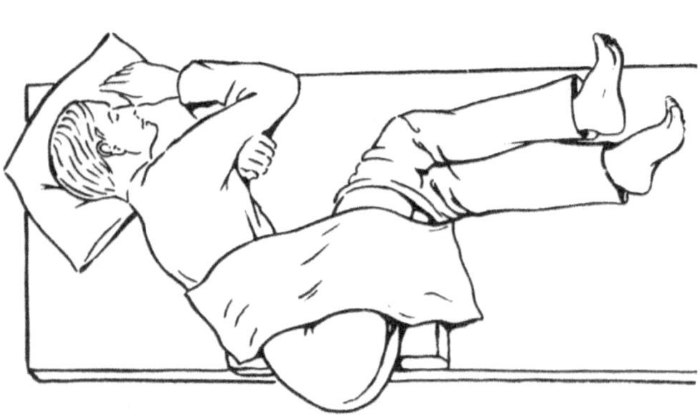

Fig. 2. The Sims's position. The patient lies on the left side with knees drawn up. The right shoulder is moved anteriorly. A small sand bag has been placed underneath the left hip.

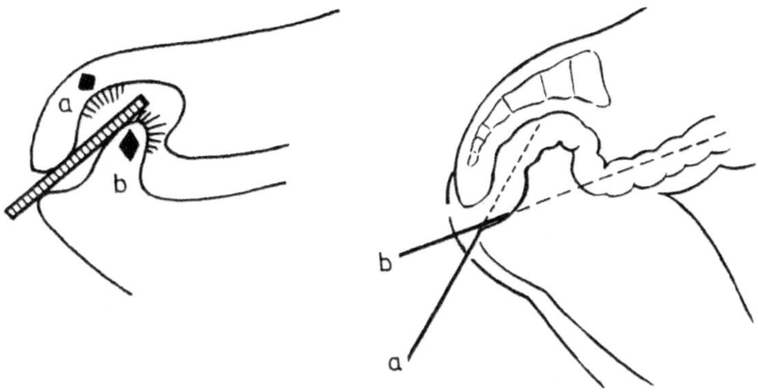

Fig. 3, a–b. "Blind areas" during protosigmoidoscopy. **a** Concavity of the sacrum. The instrument has to be pressed anteriorly against the perineum. **b** Anterior aspect of the rectosigmoid junction. The instrument is slowly withdrawn while considerable pressure is applied to the posterior aspect of the urinary bladder.

pattern of the resulting luminal collapse and mucosal fold formation than with attempts at advancing the tube by force. The distance read from the proctosigmoidoscope shaft does not always correspond to the length of bowel inspected. Occasionally, the entire sigmoid telescopes over the 30 cm length of the instrument and the descending colon is entered; more frequently, the bowel is stretched while the tube is advanced.

The depth to which the examination is ultimately carried out should be influenced by the degree of difficulties encountered, by the patient's sensitivity to pain, and by the indication for the procedure.

Air insufflation should be used sparingly, and the entire mucosal surface must be inspected by a circular motion during instrument withdrawal. The areas most difficult to visualize are the anterior wall just beyond the ventral angulation (posterior-superior aspect of the urinary bladder) and the posterior wall in the region of the lower sacrum (Fig. 3).

2.6.1.5 Indications

PS is a valuable part of preventive medicine because 80% of all colorectal tumors occur within the 30-cm reach of the instrument. Routine examination of the entire population over the age of 40 remains a desirable goal. The rectal digital examination is clearly inadequate as screening procedure for colorectal cancer and is acceptable only in the totally asymptomatic patient.

PS is indicated when blood is passed with the stool, with any change in bowel habit, and with the occurrence of any anorectal symptoms.

2.6.1.6 Contraindications

There are no contraindications to PS.

2.6.1.7 Complications

Perforation and bleeding are the most frequent complications.

Perforation of the bowel wall by the entire circumference of the instrument tip is extremely rare and can occur only with unusually vigorous manipulation. Particular caution is indicated when postoperative adhesions have caused fixation of the sigmoid in the pelvis, when the bowel wall is thinned and friable due to transmural inflammatory processes, and when the instrument is caught in a diverticulum.

Most perforations occur during excisional biopsies. This risk can be avoided by the use of forceps with a small and laterally angulated biopsy head. Forceps of this type allow the physician to pull the mucosa up and to inspect and control the biopsy site at the moment of excision. Once the forceps is closed, it should be rotated rather than pulled back immediately to disrupt tissue fibers that were not cut off. This maneuver prevents tears of the surrounding mucosa and unnecessary bleeding.

The patient must be hospitalized whenever perforation is suspected. If subsequent observations (lower abdominal pain, signs of peritoneal irritation) add to the suspicion, or if perforation is confirmed by finding free air under the diaphragm on a plain radiograph, laparotomy with closure must be performed immediately. The prognosis worsens dramatically with each hour of delay.

Bleeding occurs occasionally when a large vessel has been disrupted by the biopsy forceps. While slow venous bleeding may be expected to cease spontaneously, all arterial bleeding sites have to be attended to immediately. The site of bleeding is exposed with a large diameter endoscope; general anesthsia may be required. A combined suction-irrigation tip as well as a high-quality electrocautery unit featuring precise regulation of energy output are needed. Electrocoagulation should be performed with as low a setting as possible to avoid the danger of necrosis with late perforation (Fig. 4). Should any concern remain after arterial bleeding has been controlled with difficulty, laparotomy should be performed without hesitation. Complications of endoscopic polypectomy are discussed on p. 121.

2.6.2 Proctoscopy (Anoscopy)

Anal canal and distal rectum are examined with the proctoscope. This region is no longer collapsed after the preceding proctosigmoidoscopy but cannot be sufficiently inspected with the longer instrument.

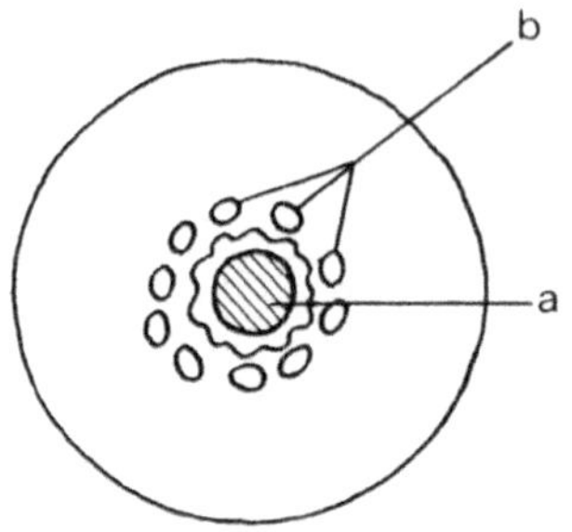

Fig. 4, a–b. Bleeding from a biopsy site. **a** Do not coagulate in the middle (*hatched area*): the wall is thinned due to loss of mucosa, and the bleeding vessels enter submucosally from the circumference. **b** Correct: multiple coagulation points surrounding the biopsy site will not miss the bleeding vessel; decreased danger of necrosis with perforation.

2.6.2.1 Instruments

Only proctoscopes with antegrade view permit adequate visualization and inspection of the circumference of the anal canal at the same level. Instruments with a lateral window are used for detailed viewing of circumscribed lesions, such as ulcers or hemorrhoids.

2.6.2.2 Preparation

Defecation is the only preparation needed when only proctoscopy is to be performed.

2.6.2.3 Postprocedure Care

There is no need for postprocedure care.

2.6.2.4 Technique

The patient assumes the same position as for PS. The instrument is introduced in a slightly posterior direction with the obturator in place to avoid pain. The obturator is then removed and the air insufflated during PS escapes. Mucus and fecal debris are removed with a moist gauze pad. The proctoscope has to be advanced and withdrawn several times for complete evaluation of the anal canal.

2.6.2.5 Indications

The same indications apply as for proctosigmoidoscopy (see Sect. 2.6.1.5). The proctoscope permits inspection of the hemorrhoidal region, allowing the injection of hemorrhoids with sclerosing solutions.

2.6.2.6 Contraindications

There are no contraindications to proctoscopy.

2.6.2.7 Complications

Marked *pain* may occur when the effect of local anesthesia, applied for fissures or stenosis, for example, begins to wane. The patient should be forewarned and be supplied with pain medication to take home.

Massive *bleeding* occurs regularly when biopsies are taken from the hemorrhoidal region. Electrocoagulation is not effective in this area, and the bleeding has to be stopped by suture ligation.

Digital examination, proctosigmoidoscopy, and proctoscopy complement each other for the comprehensive diagnosis of diseases involving the anal canal, rectum, and distal sigmoid.

References

1. OTTENJANN, R., FRIMBERGER, E., WEINGART, J., BUSSE, R.: Die Bedeutung der Rectoskopie als diagnostische und therapeutische Methode. Internist (Berlin) *17*, 209 (1976)
2. OTTO, P., EWE, K.: Atlas of Rectoskopy und Coloscopy. Berlin, Heidelberg, New York: Springer 1979

2.7
Emergency Endoscopy

H. KOCH

Hemorrhage from the upper gastrointestinal tract is among the most frequent and most dangerous emergencies encountered in the practice of internal medicine.

About 85% of all acute bleeding episodes from the entire gastrointestinal tract originate proximal to the ligament of Treitz; the remaining 15% of bleeding sites are located in the distal small intestine and colon.

The prognosis of acute gastrointestinal bleeding depends not only on the amount of blood loss, age, and general condition of the patient, but to a large extent on type and location of the bleeding lesion.

The introduction of emergency endoscopy has enabled the clinician to arrive at an exact diagnosis early, at the time of active bleeding, and to initiate specific therapy without delay.

2.7.1 Instruments

Forward-viewing instruments such as model F8 (American Cystoscope Makers, Inc., 8 Pelham Parkway, Pelham Manor, NY 10803) or GIF-HD2/03, QIF-P2 or GIF-Q (Olympus Optical Corp. of America, 2 Nevada Drive, New Hyde Park, NY 11040) are used for emergency endoscopy of the upper gastrointestinal tract. In addition, side-viewing endoscopes, such as the gastroscope GF-B2 and the duodenoscope HB2/B3 (Olympus), are needed occasionally.

When bleeding from the colon is suspected, colonoscopy is performed with the usual instruments, such as model CF-MB3, CF-LB3 or CF-IB (Olympus), model F9-S or F9-L (ACMI), or model FSS/FCS (Machida).

2.7.2 Patient Preparation

Every patient with gastrointestinal bleeding should be hospitalized without delay. *Plasma volume replacement* should begin at home or in the ambulance vehicle, if feasible, to prevent hypovolemic shock. Blood typing and cross matching of sufficient units of *blood,* obtained from the donors as recently as possible, are ordered immediately upon admission. A coagulation panel is obtained, consisting of prothrombin and partial thromboplastin time and platelet count. Pulse rate, arterial and central venous pressure, urine output, erythrocyte count, and hemoglobin and hematocrit levels are determined at regular intervals. Emergency endoscopy is the next step unless the patient is in hemorrhagic shock. Treatment of shock takes precedence over all diagnostic procedures. Direct replacement of blood loss is the preferred method. Plasma expanders, such as dextran 70 (Macrodex), are very useful until whole blood can be made available.

Even when the patient has been stabilized by aggressive shock therapy, emergency endoscopy is performed without the premedication employed for elective endoscopic examination of the upper gastrointestinal tract. Contrary to our former recommendations, we lavage the stomach with ice-water only when an initial, cursory inspection of the stomach reveals large amounts of blood or blood clots. Preparation for emergency colonoscopy consists of two to three cleansing enemas.

2.7.3 Postprocedure Care

Type of bleeding lesion and rate of blood loss dictate further therapeutic strategy. Repeated assessments of cardiovascular status and hemoglobin and hematocrit levels are part of any conservative approach. Emergency laparotomy is indicated when the site identified during endoscopy is unlikely to stop bleeding spontaneously.

2.7.4 Technique

As mentioned above, emergency endoscopy of the upper gastrointestinal tract is usually performed with forward-viewing endoscopes. The instrument is introduced with the patient lying on his left side. The esophagus is inspected carefully for varices and for evidence of esophagitis. The presence of one or more clots adherent to varices identifies the site of recent bleeding; the examiner should then proceed very cautiously to avoid reactivation of the bleeding by passage of the endoscope. Nonbleeding varices do not represent a contraindication to thorough endoscopic inspection of the stomach and duodenum.

The gastric fundus and cardia region have to be studied in detail by retroflexion of the instrument. This maneuver should not be omitted in the presence of bleeding esophageal varices since gastric varices represent an additional potential bleeding site. The importance of this observation lies in the fact that the surgical approach may have to be modified when varices are shown to bleed in both organs. The procedure for emergency colonoscopy is the same as that for elective colonoscopy.

2.7.5 Indications

Emergency endoscopy is indicated in all patients with evidence of acute bleeding from the gastrointestinal tract, such as emesis of fresh blood or coffee-ground material, melenic stools, or passage of bright red blood per rectum. When fresh blood in the stomach or rectum indicate active bleeding, emergency endoscopy must be performed immediately. On the other hand, the examination may be delayed for a few hours when no evidence of active bleeding is found (e.g., endoscopy in the morning when the patient was admitted during the night).

2.7.6 Contraindications

Hemorrhagic shock is the only contraindication to emergency endoscopy. It may even be performed in patients with coagulation disorders that would constitute a contraindication to elective endoscopic procedures. Biopsies should, of course, not be obtained under these circumstances.

2.7.7 Complications

Complications of emergency endoscopy are very infrequent. Reactivation of bleeding from esophageal varices may, however, be precipitated on rare occasions. During more than 1000 emergency endoscopies, we have observed one additional complication: irreversible cardiac arrest caused by a myocardial infarction that occurred during the endoscopic procedure.

References

1. Classen, M., Ruppin, H., Demling, L.: Emergency endoscopy in the upper gastrointestinal tract. Stomach Intestine (Jap. J.) *8*, 893 (1973)
2. Cotton, P. B., Rosenberg, M. T., Ealdram, R. P. L., Axon, A. T. R.: Early endoscopy of oesophagus, stomach, and duodenal bulb in patients with hemotemesis and melaena. Br. Med. J. *1973 II*, 505

3. DEYHLE, P., BLUM, A., RUMAGALLI, I., NÜESCH, A. J., JENNY, S.: Notfallcoloskopie. Presented at 5. Kongreß für Gastroenterologische Endoskopie der Deutschen Gesellschaft für gastroenterologische Endoskopie. Erlangen, Oktober 1973
4. KOCH, H.: Akute Magendarmblutung. Fortschr. Med. *90*, 1093 (1972)
5. PALMER, E. D.: The vigorous diagnostic approach to upper gastrointestinal tract hemorrhage. J. Am. Med. Assoc. *207*, 1477 (1969)
6. STADELMANN, O., MIEDERER, S. E., KÄUFER, E.: Emergency endoscopy in cases of acute hemorrhage of the upper gastrointestinal tract. In: Urgent endoscopy of dig. and abdominal disease, Karlsbad, 1971. Basel: Karger 1972

2.8

Therapeutic Endoscopy

P. FRÜHMORGEN/M. CLASSEN

An operation is defined as a medical procedure featuring bloody or non-bloody separation of tissue. Consequently, diagnostic endoscopy meets the criteria of this definition when biopsies are obtained. It does not appear justified, therefore, to apply the term *operative endoscopy* to procedures that are performed for theraputic reasons. We propose, instead, that such interventions be considered under the heading of *therapeutic endoscopy*.

Some of the endoscopic therapeutic procedures that are feasible today (Table 1) have not yet reached the stage of wide clinical application. We

Table 1. Capabilities of therapeutic endoscopy.

Removal of foreign bodies
Polypectomy
Removal of suture material
Papillotomy
Extraction of common bile duct stones
Laser endoscopy
Sclerosing injections of esophageal varices
Crushing of concrements
Bougienage of stenoses:
Esophagus
Common bile duct
Injection therapy:
Hemangioma
Ulcer
Electrocoagulation
Resection of inoperable malignant tumors by electrocautery
Intubation of narrowed areas, prostheses

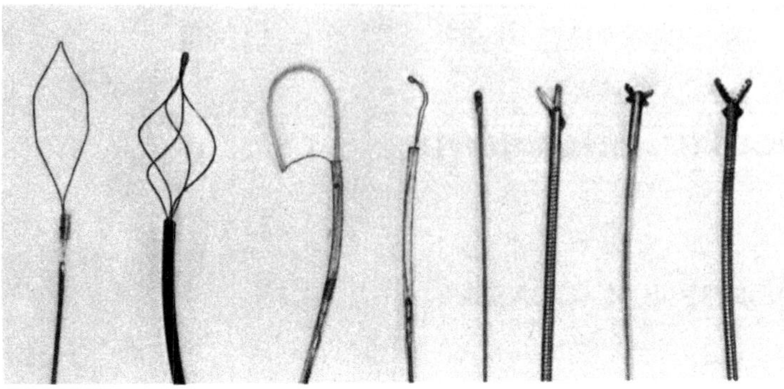

Fig. 1. Accessory instruments for foreign body removal and polypectomy; introduced through the instrumentation channel.

will, therefore, limit this discussion to those applications for which sufficient clinical experience and available instruments exist to be employed routinely by the experienced endoscopist [4].

2.8.1 Instruments

The same flexible fiber endoscopes with forward-viewing optics are used as for simple inspection of the corresponding area of the gastrointestinal tract (see pp. 59 and 87). Endoscopic papillotomy (EPT) is performed with the side-viewing duodenoscope employed for ERCP.

Foreign Body Removal. Grasping forceps of various designs, snares, and hooks (Storz, Tuttlingen, W. Germany), which are introduced through the instrumentation channel of the endoscope (Fig. 1).

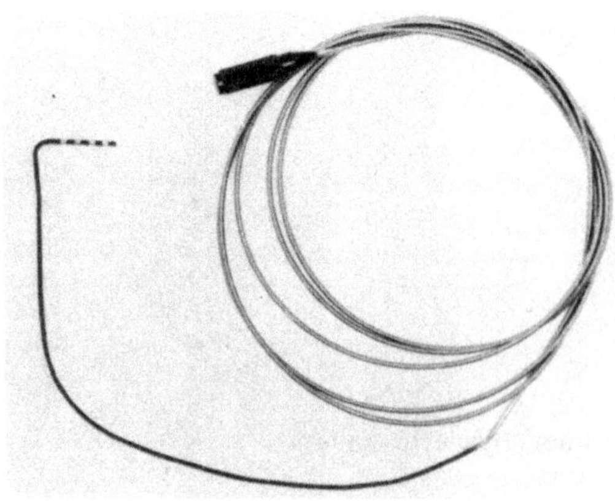

Fig. 2. Graduated, flexible measuring probe (ACMI).

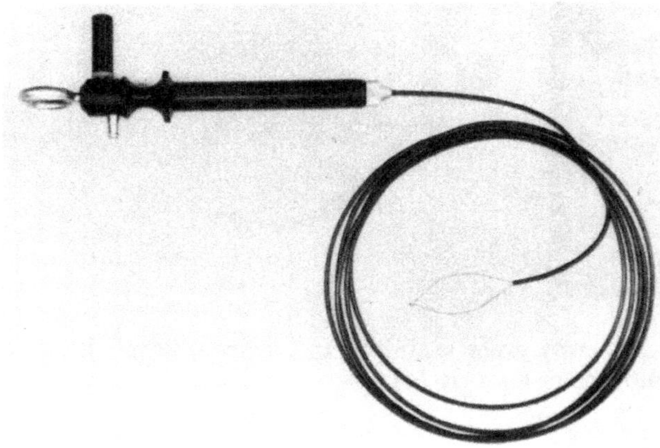

Fig. 3. Closed high-frequency diathermy snare according to Deyhle (Storz, Tuttlingen).

Polypectomy. Flexible calibration probe (ACMI); high-frequency diathermy snares (Storz, Tuttlingen, W. Germany); polyp-grasping and removal forceps; coagulation electrode; surgical high-frequency diathermy unit (Martin, Tuttlingen; Erbe, Tübingen, W. Germany; Valleylab, Boulder, CO) (Figs. 2–4).

Suture Removal. High-frequency diathermy probe according to Classen (Storz, Tuttlingen) (Fig. 5); high-frequency diathermy unit; biopsy or grasping forceps.

Endoscopic Papillotomy (EPT). Papillotome according to Demling and Classen (Storz, Tuttlingen) (Fig. 6); papillotome according to Sohma (Olympus); Dormia basket (Storz, Tuttlingen; Olympus); high-frequency diathermy unit.

Laser Coagulation. Two different energy sources are currently avail-

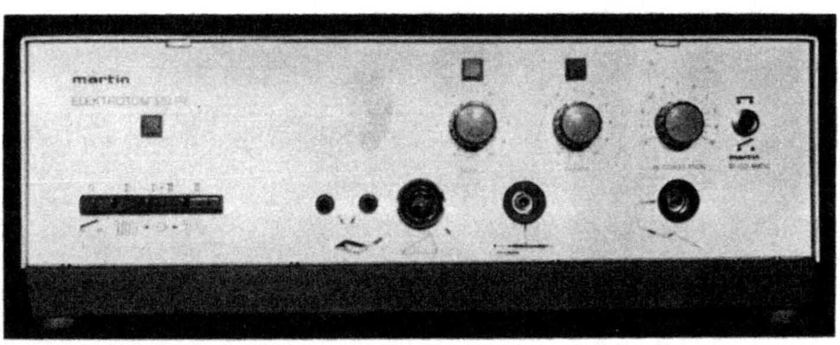

Fig. 4. High-frequency electrosurgical (diathermy) unit: Elektrotom 170 RF (Martin, Tuttlinger).

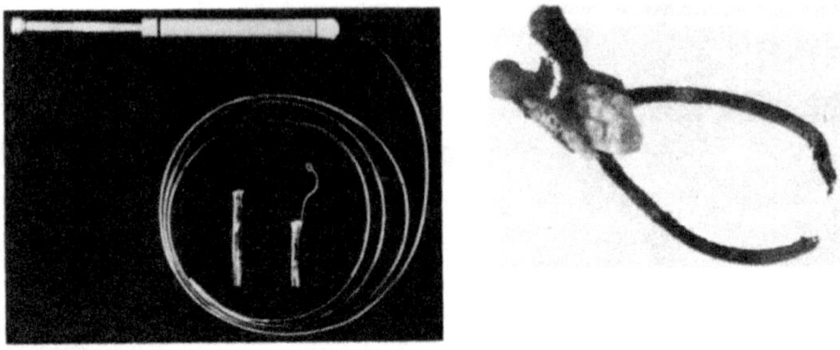

Fig. 5. High-frequency diathermy probe according to Classen (Storz, Tuttlingen) (left); removed suture with intact knot (right).

able for photocoagulation of bleeding and potentially bleeding lesions in the gastrointestinal tract; the argon ion laser (model 770; Spectra Physics, Mountain View, CA), (Fig. 7) and the neodymium-YAG laser (model mediLas; Messerschmitt-Boelkow-Blohm, Munich-Ottobrunn) (Fig. 8). Both are adaptable to endoscopic use via a fully flexible light transmission bundle. The bundle for the former can be used with any available endoscope, while the neodymium-YAG laser requires an endoscope specially modified for this purpose.

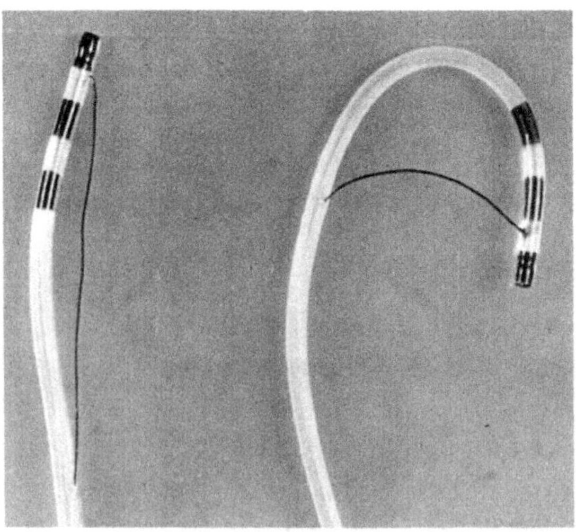

Fig. 6. Papillotome according to Demling and Classen (Storz, Tuttlingen).

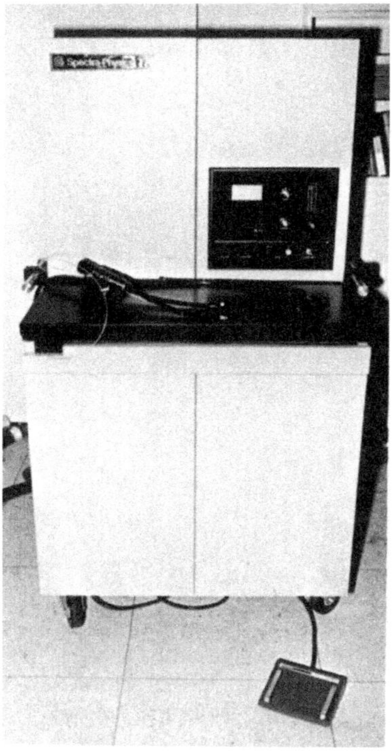

Fig. 7. Argon laser coagulator (model 770, Spectra-Physics, Mountain View, CA).

2.8.2 Patient Preparation

The same as for the corresponding diagnostic endoscopic procedure (pp. 61 and 90). General anesthesia for children and patients suffering from mental disorders. The location of radiopaque foreign bodies should be verified immediately prior to the attempt at endoscopic extraction because they frequently change position or may even have been passed per rectum in the meantime. The preparation for laser coagulation of bleeding lesions is no different than that for emergency endoscopy (p. 108).

2.8.3 Postprocedure Care

In-hospital observation for 24 h, depending on individual circumstances; 48 h or more after EPT and laser coagulation.

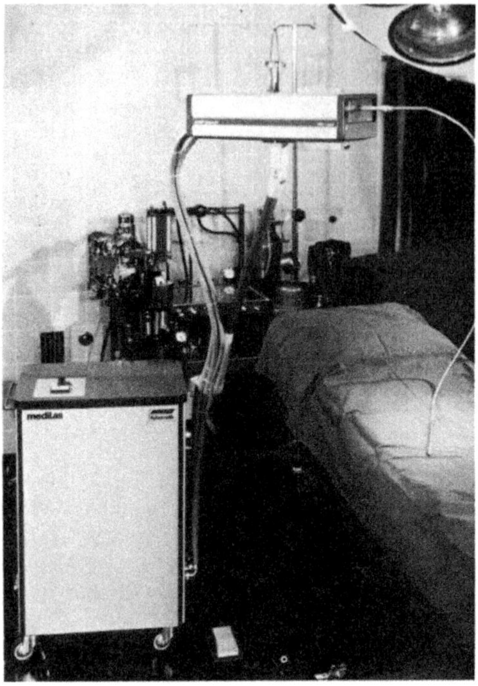

Fig. 8. Neodymium-YAG laser coagulator (model mediLas, Messerschmitt-Bölkow-Blohm, Munich).

2.8.4 Technique

2.8.4.1 Foreign Body Removal

The principle of the removal of foreign bodies arrested in the gastrointestinal tract [22,26,27] is the peroral or peranal extraction across physiologic or pathologic areas of luminal narrowing (Table 2). The initial approach should be expectant observation for 1 or 2 weeks since 80%–90% of all foreign bodies are passed spontaneously. Pointed objects and those with sharp edges must be extracted immediately because of the danger of perforation [25]. Foreign bodies greater than 2 cm in diameter or longer than 5 cm should also be removed without delay since they rarely pass the pylorus. Small objects can be grasped with the usual biopsy forceps, coins preferably with a modified Jackson forceps (jaws converted to a saw-tooth pattern), and large foreign bodies with the snare used for endoscopic polypectomy. The extraction is carried out under direct observation by simultaneous withdrawal of foreign body and endoscope. Injury during extraction of sharp objects, such as razor blades, can be avoided by use of a plastic sheath surrounding the endoscope. As soon as the foreign body is grasped the sheath is advanced beyond the instrument tip, thus protecting the gastrointestinal mucosa from damage. Tricho- and phytobezoars [22]

Table 2. Therapy of foreign bodies by fiberoptic endoscopy (n = 106).

I. Mobilization or extraction (esophagus)	
Prune pit	2
Cellulose bolus	1
Food bolus	5
II. Extraction (stomach, duodenum, choledochus)	
Coins	48
Hair barette	1
Tip of nasogastric tube	1
Intestinal biopsy tube	1
Wire (15 cm)	1
T tube	1
Polypectomy snare	1
Teaspoon	3
Ring	2
Food residue	8
Glass ball	1
Suture material	19
Nail	6
Battery	1
Watch	1
III. Extraction (colon)	
Enema tip	1
Transintestinal tube	1
Suture material	1

and impacted food boluses can be broken up with the biopsy forceps into pieces that will pass through the gastrointestinal tract.

2.8.4.2 Polypectomy

Endoscopic ablation with the high-frequency diathermy snare [2,5,7,13, 9,11,30] is the method of choice for dealing with polypoid lesions.

High-frequency currents [28] of around 1.7 MHz induce local heat (Nernst's law) without danger of nerve stimulation or electric shock. The tissue is severed by the combined action of cutting (sinusoidal) and coagulation (spark gap) current. The commercially available units can deliver both types of current; experience has shown the ratio of 1:1, better in our opinion is coagulation current, to be optimal. The current is generated at 500–700 V. Current flow decreases markedly as the tissue becomes dehydrated during ablation; this reduces the risk of thermal damage to the deeper layers of the viscus. Patients with cardiac pacemakers should not undergo polypectomy with high-frequency diathermy current because of the danger of electric interference [23].

The selection of the optimal current setting has to be individualized and requires considerable experience. It is advisable to begin with a low dial setting [e.g., step 3 on the Erbotom (Erbe) or the Elektrotom 170 RF (Martin)] and short impulse duration. Current delivery is then slowly increased under constant observation of the cutting and coagulating effect until the polyp is severed. The dial setting on the surgical high-frequency diathermy unit bears little relationship to the energy actually delivered by the polypectomy snare because the two are not linearly related and because current delivery depends on the variable tissue resistance and on the type of unit used.

After size and shape of the polyp have been assessed, the snare is slipped over the head of the lesion and adjusted to surround its base. Next, the snare is pulled back cautiously until the polyp acquires a dusky, cyanotic coloration. Current is then applied while the snare is tightened further, pulling the lesion toward the lumen to avoid thermal injury to the deep tissue layers and to the surrounding mucosa (Fig. 9).

The polyp is recovered with a biopsy forceps, a grasping forceps, or by aspiration. The size of the lesion can be measured before ablation with a graduated measuring probe introduced through the instrumentation channel or after the polyp has been delivered to the outside. Several polyps can be removed in this fashion during single passage of the endoscope. We recommend that antral and duodenal polyps be biopsied before polypectomy because they occasionally escape recovery.

Note:

a) Attach the indifferent electrode near the site of polypectomy (thigh) with good contact over a large skin area.
b) Do not turn on the high-frequency current as long as the snare touches the bowel wall or metal parts of the endoscope.

2.8.4.3 Removal of Sutures

Seromuscular sutures consisting of nonresorbable material such as silk and polyester fiber (Mersilene; Ethicon Co., Sommerville, NJ) are visible in about 10% of patients who have undergone gastric operations. Suture ulcers develop in about one out of ten of these cases, causing dyspeptic symptoms and slow bleeding [16,27,29]. The suture can sometimes be removed with the biopsy forceps, but the physician should be alert to the possibility of narrowing the anastomotic lumen in cases where the suture

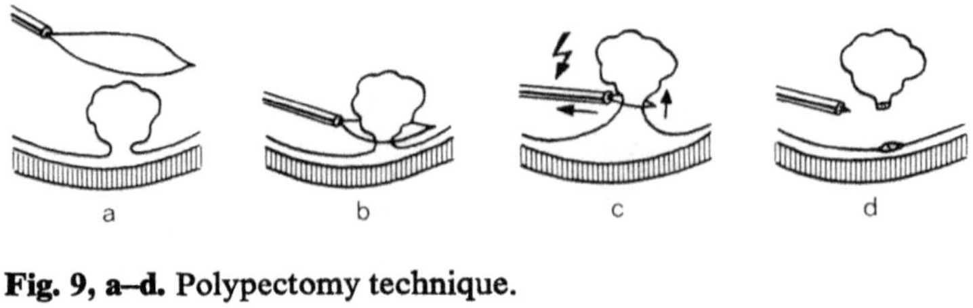

Fig. 9, a–d. Polypectomy technique.

is continuous. Alternatively, the thread is cut with a special high-frequency probe and extracted by forceps [6].

2.8.4.4 Endoscopic Papillotomy (EPT)

When diagnostic ERCP demonstrates papillary stenosis or bile stasis due to narrowing of the distal common duct, the operator may proceed immediately with introducing the papillotome into the common bile duct [17,20,31]. Position and spatial orientation of the papillotome are checked endoscopically, as well as radiologically, following injection of contrast material into the duct. Accidental cannulation and incision of the pancreatic duct is dangerous and is to be strictly avoided. Next, the roof of the papilla is incised by high-frequency current to the point of transition to the duodenal wall or beyond. The length of the incision depends on type and extent of the obstructing lesion, such as tumor size or dimensions of a common duct stone. The choice of the power output setting is similar to that described on p. 118. Low power is used initially (mixed current: step 4 for cutting; step 2 for coagulation) with brief impulse duration; increases in power setting and delivery time depend on the result obtained. High power settings applied without frequent interruption lead to completion of the incision within seconds, allowing insufficient time for careful tailoring of incision length to the individual patient. Incisions extending far into the duodenal wall are dangerous because of the unpredictable course of the retroduodenal artery. Common duct stones pass spontaneously in 73% of our patients after EPT; the rest are extracted endoscopically with a Dormia basket.

2.8.4.5 Laser Coagulation

Photocoagulation of bleeding and potentially bleeding lesions [14,15,19,18] is carried out during or immediately following the diagnostic endoscopic procedure. The laser beam is applied for a few seconds under direct visual control while the physician's eye is protected by a special filter. Exensive experience with endoscopic techniques is an absolute prerequisite, particularly with the neodymium-YAG laser, which carries an increased risk of perforation.

Tissue penetration and depth of coagulation necrosis are dictated by the wavelength of the laser beam, the energy output setting chosen, impulse duration, and the type of lesion being coagulated. It should be noted that the achievement of comparable coagulation requires a four to five times higher energy delivery by the neodymium-YAG compared to the argon laser. With a loss of 10%–20% during transmission, the energy delivered at the tip of the instrument varies between 10 and 15 W with the argon and between 60 and 100 W with the neodymium-YAG laser. The selective absorption of the argon beam in the red part of the spectrum (blood and blood vessels) appears to give this modality an advantage over the neodymium-YAG laser. This holds true only if the bleeding lesion can be kept free of blood during laser application. A CO_2 gas jet is routinely integrated into the laser delivery system for this purpose.

2.8.5 Indications

Foreign Body Removal. Objects that cannot pass through the gastrointestinal tract due to their size or shape.

Polypectomy. All polypoid lesions must be removed for diagnostic reasons since the entire lesion must be examined histologically to rule out a malignant process (Tables 3 and 4).

Removal of Sutures. Suture ulcer and slow bleeding from the point of suture penetration through the mucosa.

Endoscopic Papillotomy. Stenosis of the papilla of Vater; choledocholithiasis in patients carrying high surgical risk factors.

Laser Coagulation. Bleeding as well as nonbleeding vascular malformations; bleeding erosions, ulcers and varices; iatrogenic bleeding following large-particle gastric biopsy or polypectomy; and bleeding inoperable tumors. Diffuse mucosal bleeding, in ulcerative colitis, for example, is not currently considered an indication for photocoagulation.

The value and clinical applicability of this method cannot yet be fully assessed. The equipment is expensive (80 000—100 000 DM) and is relatively immobile because of connections to cooling water and to three-phase current.

2.8.6 Contraindications

The same as those for the corresponding endoscopic examination (pp. 66 and 97) with emphasis on the presence of hemorrhagic diatheses.

Table 3. Histologic diagnosis of polyps removed from the upper gastrointestinal tract (n = 249).

Hyperplasiogenous polyp	150
Hyperplastic polyp	26
Adenomata	2
Peutz-Jeghers polyp	16
Cronkhite-Canada polyp	1
Carcinoma	10
Lipoma	1
Ectopic pancreas	8
Hemangioma	3
Neurinoma/neurofibroma	6
Borderline lesion	3
Pseudopolyp after Billroth II	5
Polypoid or normal mucosa	18

Table 4. Histologic diagnosis of polyps removed from the lower gastrointestinal tract (n = 1286).

Adenoma	
Tubular	727
Tubular-villous	125
Villous	66
With severe atypia	38
Hyperplastic polyp	205
Carcinoma	76
Cronkhite-Canada Polyp	1
Peutz-Jeghers Polyp	27
Pseudopolyp	5
Carcinoid	1
Juvenile polyp	10
Lipoma	4
Angiofibroma	1

2.8.7 Complications

2.8.7.1 Polypectomy

Bleeding. Bleeding may occur with insufficient electrocoagulation of the remaining polyp stalk during polypectomy and with mechanical polyp removal without use of high-frequency diathermy current. Low-grade bleeding will cease spontaneously but should be observed through the colonoscope. Careful electro- or laser coagulation, or surgical intervention should be undertaken for brisk bleeding. With polyps on a long stalk, a 2–3 mm stump should be left behind, which can be "lassoed" again with the polypectomy snare in case bleeding occurs. A poll of endoscopists in West Germany revealed the risk of severe hemorrhage to be 2.24% following 7365 polypectomies [10].

Perforation. This danger arises when the polyp base is greater than 3 cm in diameter and in those cases in which the colonic wall itself is pulled into the polypectomy snare (Fig. 10d, f).

We cannot recommend the submucosal *injection of physiologic saline* around the polyp for providing heat insulation because this makes the polypectomy more difficult by widening the polyp base (Fig. 10g). Furthermore, inadvertent injection of the polyp itself cannot always be avoided (Fig. 10h). When the polypectomy is then carried through this fluid depot, the polyp may be only partially removed, risking recurrence of an adenomatous or malignant lesion. The poll of endoscopists mentioned earlier revealed the risk of perforation to be 0.34% during 7365 polypectomies [10].

Gas Explosion. The combination of a combustible gas mixture in the bowel lumen and the occasional occurrence of sparks caused by the

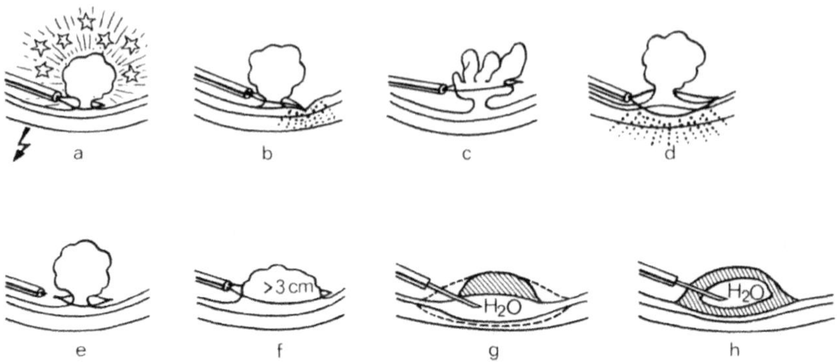

Fig. 10, a–h. Possible complications during polypectomy: **a** gas explosion; **b** thermal damage to the mucosa; **c** incomplete polypectomy; **d** colonic wall pulled into the snare; **e** snare fracture; **f** polyp base greater than 3 cm; **g** submucosal injection of physiologic saline; **h** polypectomy through a fluid depot.

high voltage of the high-frequency current at the active electrode provides the setting for explosions (Fig. 10a). Hydrogen gas and methane, both produced almost exclusively in the colonic lumen, can form explosive mixtures with oxygen if present above certain concentrations. There are several reports of explosions during electrosurgical operations in the colon, including polypectomy [1,3,21,24]. We investigated this problem by measuring colonic intraluminal hydrogen and methane concentrations with three different types of patient preparation: group 1, no colon cleansing, stimulation of gas production by feeding beans; group 2, no cleansing and no stimulation of gas production; group 3, colon cleansing by diet, magnesium sulfate, and enemas. Hydrogen and methane were determined by gas chromatography. We found the critical explosive concentration of both gases to be 4 vol.%. This concentration was exceeded in groups 1 and 2, but the values in group 3 were less than 0.01 vol.%. We conclude, therefore, that there is no danger of explosion during electrosurgery within the colon as long as the organ has been evacuated thoroughly of bacteria and their food-derived substrates [12]. However, when colon cleansing is omitted or when gas formation is stimulated, hydrogen and methane concentration may exceed the critical limit. We forego insufflation of the colon with an inert gas, such as CO_2, for electrosurgical procedures when the organ has been cleansed thoroughly by our method (p. 90). Using mannitol solution (sweet lavage) for bowel preparation there was, however, recently a first report of a fatal colonic explosion during colonoscopic polypectomy [32].

Snare fracture at the soldering point is the result of a mechanical defect or of faulty technique. The polyp should then be removed with a new snare and should be recovered together with the broken snare (Fig. 10e).

Incomplete polypectomy, particularly of multilobulated lesions, and *thermal damage* to the mucosa hidden behind the polyp by the apex of the snare can be avoided when sufficient care is exercised (Fig. 10b, c).

2.8.7.2 Endoscopic Papillotomy

The complication rate of EPT is about 8%, representing mainly acute bleeding and cholangitis. The usual cause of the latter is impaction of a stone in the papilla of Vater following an imcomplete EPT. Most complications manifest themselves within the first 24 h after the procedure. The worldwide mortality rate is 0.9%.

2.8.7.3 Laser Coagulation

Possible complications are perforation and increased bleeding due to rupture of a blood vessel. The expected incidence of complications at a time when this procedure becomes widely employed cannot be estimated because it currently is used only by a very few, highly experienced physicians. While the Erlangen group was unsuccessful on 3 of 271 occasions but encountered no complications [14,15], the Munich group [19,20] reported a perforation rate of 1% and recurrent bleeding in 17% of 204 patients so treated.

References

1. BECKER, G. L.: Prevention of gas explosions in the large bowel during electro-surgery. Surg. Gynecol. Obstet. *97*, 463 (1953)
2. BLACKWOOD, W. D., SILVIS, S. E.: Gastroscopic elextrosurgery. Gastroenterology *3*, 305 (1971)
3. CARTER, H. G.: Explosion in the colon during electrodesiccation of polyps. Am. J. Surg. *84*, 515 (1952)
4. CLASSEN, M., FRÜHMORGEN, P.: Operative endoscopy in the gastrointestinal tract. Acta Hepato-gastroenterol. (Stuttg.) *19*, 124 (1972)
5. CLASSEN, M., ZEUS, J., DEMLING, L.: Endoskopische Polypektomie im oberen Verdauungstrakt. Leber Magen Darm *3*, 163 (1973)
6. CLASSEN, M., RÖSCH, W., FRÜHMORGEN, P., SEUBERTH, K., DEMLING, L.: Operative endoscopy: A diathermy-hook for cutting of non-absorbable material. Endoscopy *6*, 42 (1974)
7. DEYHLE, P., SEUBERTH, K., JENNY, S., DEMLING, L.: Endoscopic polypectomy in the proximal colon. Endoscopy *2*, 103 (1971)
8. DEYHLE, P., LARGIADER, F., JENNY, S., FUMAGALLI, I.: A method for endoscopic electroresection of sessile colonic polypes. Endoscopy *5*, 38 (1973)
9. FRÜHMORGEN, P.: Operative Endoskopie im Kolon. Fortschr. Med. *16*, 685 (1973)
10. FRÜHMORGEN, P., DEMLING, L.: Complications of diagnostic and therapeutic colonoscopy in the Federal Republic of Germany. Results of an Inquiry. Endoscopy *2*, 146 (1979)
11. FRÜHMORGEN, P., DEMLING, L.: Koloskopische Polypektomie. Dtsch. Med. Wochenschr. *98*, 1455 (1973)

12. Frühmorgen, P., Joachim, G.: Gas chromatographic analyses of intestinal gas to clarify the question of inert gas insufflation in electrosurgical endoscopy. Endoscopy *8*, 133 (1976)
13. Frühmorgen, P., Zeus, J., Demling, L.: Endoskopisch-operative Behandlung polypoider Läsionen des Dickdarms. Leber Magen Darm *3*, 166 (1973)
14. Frühmorgen, P., Bodem, F., Reidenbach, H. D., Kaduk, B., Demling, L.: Endoscopic laser coagulation of bleeding gastrointestinal lesions with report of the first therapeutic application in man. Gastrointest. Endosc. *2*, 139 (1977)
15. Frühmorgen, P., Bodem, F., Reidenbach, H. D., Kaduk, B., Demling, L.: Endoscopic photocoagulation by laser irradiation in the gastrointestinal tract of man. Acta Hepato-Gastroenterol. (Stuttg.) *25*, 1 (1978)
16. Gear, M. W. L., Dowling, B. L.: Suture–line ulcer after gastric surgery caused by non-absorbable suture material. Br. J. Surg. *57*, 356 (1970)
17. Kawai, K., Nakaima, M., Kimoto, K., Sugawara, K., Fukumoto, K.: Endoscopic sphincterotomy of the ampulla of Vater. Endoscopy *7*, 30 (1975)
18. Kiefhaber, P.: Neodym-YAG-laser. In: Operative endoscopy (In preparation)
19. Kiefhaber, P., Nath, G., Moritz, K., Kreitmair, A.: Der Einsatz des Neodym-YAG-lasers bei der endoskopischen Blutstillung im Rahmen der Notfallendoskopie. In: Fortschritte der gastroenterologischen Endoskopie. Lindner, H. (Ed.), Vol. VIII, p. 226. Baden-Baden: Witzstrock 1977
20. Koch, H., Rösch, W., Schaffner, O., Demling, L.: Endoscopic papillotomy. Gastroenterology *73*, 1393 (1977)
21. Levy, E. I.: Explosions during lower bowel electrosurgery. Am. J. Surg. *88*, 754 (1954)
22. Lukash, W. M., Fornes, M. F., Johnson, R. B.: Gastric bezoars. Gastroenterology *58*, 1070 (1970)
23. Mauser, R.: Störeinflüsse auf Herzschrittmacher durch Elektrochirurgiegeräte. Elektronik *20*, 199 (1971)
24. Moutier, M. F.: Un nouveau cas d'explosion intrarectale au cours d'une electrocoagulation. Arch. Mal. Appar. Dig. *35*, 240 (1946)
25. Perelman, H.: Toothpick perforation of the gastrointestinal tract. J. Abdom. Surg. *4*, 51 (1962)
26. Rösch, W., Classen, M.: Fiberendoscopic foreign body removal from the upper GI-tract. Endoscopy *4*, 193 (1972)
27. Rösch, W., Classen, M.: Fiberendoskopische Entfernung von Fremdkörpern aus dem Verdauungstrakt. Leber Magen Darm *3*, 169 (1973)
28. v. Seeman, V.: Allgemeine und spezielle Elektrochirurgie. Berlin: Springer 1932
29. Small, W. P., Smith, A. N., Ruchley, C. V., Falconer, C. W. A., Sircus, W., McManus, J. P. A., Bruce, Sir J: The continuing problem of jejunal ulcer. Am. J. Surg. *121*, 541 (1971)
30. Tsuneoka, K., Uchida, T.: Endoscopic polypectomy of the stomach. Gastrointest. Endosc. *11*, 183 (1970)
31. Zimmon, D. S., Falkenstein, D. B., Kessler, R. E.: Endoscopic papillotomy for choledocholithiasis. N. Engl. J. Med. *293*, 1181 (1975)
32. Bigard, M. A., Gaucher, P., Lasalle, C.: Fatal colonic explosion during colonoscopic polypectomy. Gastroenterology *77*, 1307 (1979)

2.9

Blind Aspiration Biopsy

W. RÖSCH

Until recently, blind aspiration biopsy was the leading method for the morphologic diagnosis of gastrointestinal diseases. The advent of fully flexible fiber endoscopes has greatly decreased the need and, therefore, the importance of this approach. Today, blind gastric biopsy should no longer be employed and is only of historic importance. While blind esophageal biopsy never found wide clinical acceptance, blind small intestinal biopsy, obtained distal to the ligament of Treitz, remains the method of choice when the presence of a malabsorption syndrome is suspected.

2.9.1 Instruments

The aspiration biopsy instrument developed by Henning and Heinkel (Figs. 1 and 2) was specifically designed for obtaining mucosal particles from the esophagus and stomach and found wide acceptance. Heinkel modified this tube by adding a more flexible tip to facilitate antral biopsies under fluoroscopic control. All biopsy instruments feature a capsule containing a circular knife that can be moved back and forth in a hollow cylinder severing the mucosal particle aspirated through the biopsy port. The size of the specimen is dictated by the size of the circular hole in the capsule; unfortunately, the manufacturers recently have tended to decrease this aperture.

Intestinal biopsy instruments are available that allow multiple particles to be obtained from different areas (Quinton-Rubin Hydraulic Biopsy Tube, Quinton Instrument Co., Seattle, WA). The tube contains two channels, one for hydraulic operation of the knife, the other for flushing the mucosal specimen. The disadvantage of this instrument is that it takes relatively long to reach its proper position. We use the modified Watson-Camus intestinal

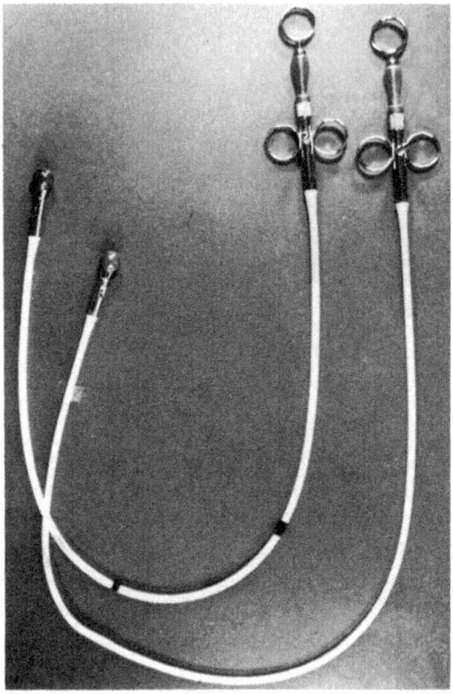

Fig. 1. Gastric aspiration biopsy instrument according to Henning and Heinkel.

biopsy tube (Watson-Classen Probe; Storz, Tuttlingen), which can be placed within a few minutes (Fig. 3). The biopsy knife is activated by a spring and held open by a retaining bolt. Once in the intestine, the knife is released by applying a vacuum of about 350 mm Hg. The tube has to be removed after each such excision attempt. This is a distinct disadvantage when the maneuver is unsuccessful in obtaining a biopsy particle.

The original intestinal biopsy capsule of Crosby and Kugler [1] also utilizes a spring-loaded cutting knife that is released following aspiration of mucosa through the biopsy port. The Quinton-Rubin hydraulic tube [2] is the most popular instrument in use because multiple biopsies can be obtained from the esophagus to the terminal ileum during a single intubation. Each biopsy particle is delivered to the outside by a high-pressure stream of saline, and the knife returns to its resting position when the pressure is released.

Several suggestions have recently been made for facilitating the placement of intestinal biopsy instruments. The tube can be introduced together with a fiberoptic endoscope and then grasped with the biopsy forceps to be guided through the pylorus under visual control. Prout [6] described a different method whereby the Crosby biopsy capsule is covered with a rubber jacket and a radiopaque arterial catheter is threaded through the instru-

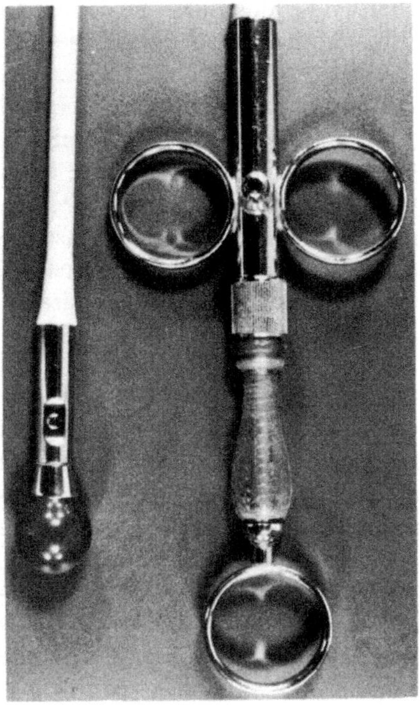

Fig. 2. Enlarged view of parts of Fig. 1.

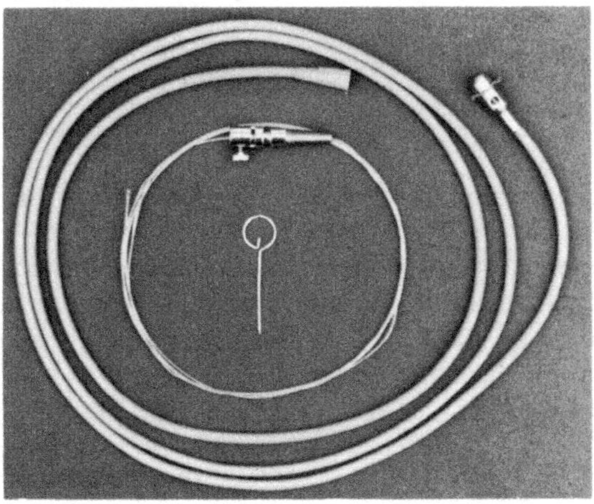

Fig. 3. Small intestinal biopsy instrument according to Watson and Classen.

mentation channel of an end-viewing fiberoptic endoscope. The endoscope is passed through the pylorus, pushing the capsule ahead toward the duodenojejunal flexure.

Enteroscopy is rarely used for sampling of the small bowel mucosa. In many centers, however, guided biopsies are routinely obtained from the third portion of the duodenum with the side-viewing duodenoscope when anatomic abnormalities impede passage of the aspiration biopsy tube into its proper position. The pathognomonic changes of Whipple's disease are already present in the duodenal bulb, while sampling of the proximal jejunum remains the preferred approach to the diagnosis of celiac disease.

2.9.2 Patient Preparation

No special preparation is necessary for aspiration biopsies. The patient should be fasting. Food particles may occlude the biopsy port in the presence of gastric outlet obstruction. No premedication is required and topical anesthesia of the pharynx can frequently be omitted.

A normal coagulation panel (prothrombin time, partial thromboplastin time, and platelet count) is an indispensable prerequisite for any aspiration biopsy because some bleeding is expected to occur with the excision of biopsy particles which are up to 5×5 mm in size. If it is planned to perform a blind gastric aspiration biopsy without fluroscopic control, then an esophagogram should be obtained first to rule out the presence of large diverticula.

2.9.3 Postprocedure Care

No special measures are required after aspiration biopsies other than advising the patient of the risk of bleeding. The patient should immediately contact his physician when hematemesis or melena occur after aspiration biopsy performed on an outpatient basis. Written consent is required in most instituions, which informs the patient of possible complications and the therapeutic measures that may become necessary.

2.9.4 Technique

The site of *blind esophageal biopsy* is the distal esophagus, 30–38 cm from the incisor teeth. Adequate material, containing mucosa and muscularis mucosae, is obtained when 250 mm Hg of negative pressure are applied for 3–5 s (specific instructions accompanying each biopsy instrument should be followed). The average thickness is 0.45 mm. Attempts should be made to obtain several particles by rotating the biopsy capsule, particularly since not every biopsy maneuver is successful.

Blind gastric biopsies, preferably from the greater curvature, are obtained with the capsule advanced 45–50 cm beyond the incisor teeth. The axial position of the biopsy capsule within the stomach can be determined without fluoroscopy since biopsy port and external connector for aspiration remain in the same plane. The necessary vacuum can be produced with any tight-fitting syringe but is more easily obtained by a vacuum pump equipped with a manometer. A negative pressure of 350–400 mm Hg, applied for 3–5 s, is required. The particles measure 0.7–1.0 mm in thickness. Fluoroscopic tube placement is necessary when the antrum is to be biopsied.

Fluoroscopic verification of the tube position in the anterior-posterior and lateral plane is required for *small intestinal biopsy* (Fig. 4). The stiffening wire of the Watson-Classen instrument allows the biopsy capsule to be positioned in the prepyloric antrum without excess slack in the stomach. The wire is then partially withdrawn and the biopsy tube actively advanced into the duodenum (Fig. 5). At this point, the stiffening wire is removed completely. When the biopsy capsule has reached the desired position, a negative pressure of 350–400 mm Hg is applied with the patient sitting and bending forward.

The biopsy particle is first examined with a stereoscopic microscope at a magnification of ×10–×20. The normal duodenum and proximal jejunum show finger-, leaf-, and ridge-shaped villi that measure between 200 μm and 700 μm in height. Shortened villi give an appearance similar to that of the brain surface. This pattern is termed "convoluted mucosa," indicating partial villous atrophy. The mucosa appears completely flat with

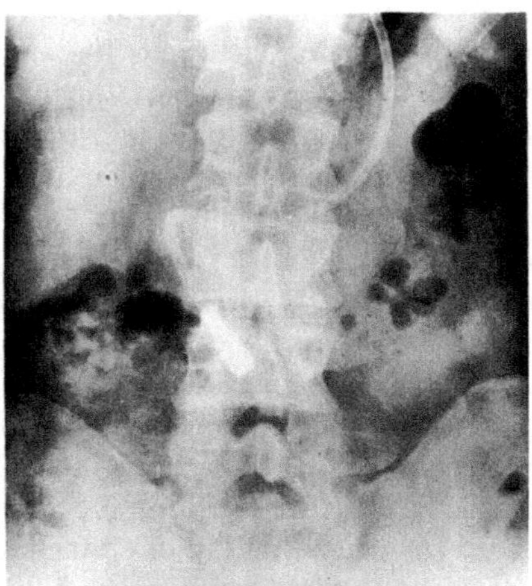

Fig. 4. Biopsy capsule in duodenum.

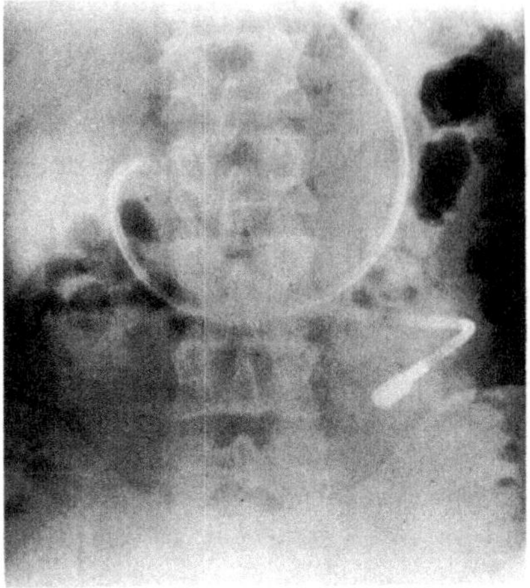

Fig. 5. Biopsy capsule in correct position, distal to the ligament of Treitz.

the total villous atrophy regularly present in untreated celiac disease. The biopsy particle is then placed, mucosal side up, on a piece of nylon mesh or Gelfoam and submitted for histologic study.

2.9.5 Indications

Blind aspiration biopsy of the esophagus has not yet found wide acceptance in clinical practice, mainly because the correlation between clinical symptomatology and histologic evidence of esophagitis is weak [7]. More recent results, however, raise the hope that this method may reveal early changes of esophagitis, such as basal cell hyperplasia, before macroscopic changes appear [3]. Ottenjann [4] has proposed the term "hyperregeneratory esophagopathy" for these histologic changes, in analogy to celiac disease. Esophageal aspiration biopsy is the preferred method for research in this area since the full epithelial thickness is obtained while the endoscopic biopsy forceps yields only the superficial layers of the mucosal epithelium.

The value of gastric aspiration biopsies decreased greatly when serial biopsies, obtained endoscopically along the greater and lesser curvature, revealed that gastritis is by no means a diffuse lesion. Rather, gastritis frequently is focal, and extension from the pylorus toward the cardia needs to be distinguished from the reverse process [5]. Furthermore, the appearance of biopsies obtained without visual control does not correlate with the functional capacity of the gastric mucosa [8]. Thus, the only remaining indication for gastric aspiration biopsy is the suspected presence of diffuse mucosal hyperplasia where large particles are needed for determination of epithelial thickness. Even this indication is disappearing with the development of the "large particle" biopsy technique by which a hyperplastic fold can be removed *in toto* with the diathermy snare.

Small intestinal biopsy is indicated when intestinal inflammatory processes are suspected, particularly in the presence of symptoms suggesting malabsorption. All types of sprue, intestinal lymphangiectasia, Whipple's disease, giardiasis with nodular lymphoid hyperplasia, and occasionally, Crohn's disease require histologic verification. *Giardia lamblia* is easily discovered on smears made from the surface of the mucosal particle, analogous to imprint cytology. Biochemical analysis of biopsy material for congenital or acquired oligosaccharidase deficiencies is primarily of scientific interest and is rarely needed for clinical purposes.

2.9.6 Contraindications

The main contraindications to aspiration biopsy of the proximal gastrointestinal tract are hemorrhagic diatheses and suspected portal hypertension with esophageal, fundic, or duodenal varices. The risk of perforation is higher in children with celiac disease; therefore, less vacuum should be applied when obtaining the biopsy.

2.9.7 Complications

Blind aspiration biopsy procedures carry a higher complication rate than biopsies procured through the endoscope. No complications have been reported so far with esophageal aspiration biopsy. The bleeding rate after gastric biopsy is 0.26% with an even lower incidence of perforation. The latter complication is essentially limited to intestinal biopsy in the presence of severe intestinal disease (0.01%–0.05%). The intestinal biopsy capsule may occasionally remain attached to the mucosa due to incomplete excision of the particle, or it may resist withdrawal from the duodenum. These problems usually resolve with time, without the need for active intervention.

References

1. Crosby, W. H., Kugler, H. W.: Intraluminal biopsy of the small intestine: The intestinal biopsy capsule. Am. J. Dig. Dis. *2*, 236 (1957)
2. Flick, A. L., Quinton, W. E., Rubin, C. E.: A peroral hydraulic biopsy tube for multiple sampling at any level of the gastrointestinal tract. Gastroenterology *40*, 120 (1961)
3. Ismail-Beigi, F., Horton, P. F., Pope, C. E.: Histological consequences of gastroesophageal reflux in man. Gastroenterology *58*, 163 (1970)

4. Ottenjann, R., Gruner, H. J., Strauch, M.: Endoskopisch-bioptische Befunde bei Refluxösophagitis. Leber Magen Darm *2*, 48 (1972a)
5. Ottenjann, R., Bartelheimer, W., Beck, K., Kanzler, G., Elster, K.: Die blinde Aspirationsbiopsie der Magenschleimhaut. Kritik der Methode. Dtsch. Med. Wochenschr. *97*, 221 (1972b)
6. Prout, B. J.: A rapid technique of obtaining a jejunal biopsy using a Crosby capsule and a gastrointestinal fiberscope. ??? *15*, 571 (1974)
7. Rösch, W., Stadelmann, O., Ottenjann, R.: Die blinde Ösophagobiopsie —eine risikoarme Untersuchungsmethode. Endoscopy *1*, 21 (1969)
8. Stadelmann, O., Elster, K., Miederer, S. E., Kaip, E.: Gastritis und peptisches Geschwür. In: Peptisches Geschwür. Demling, L., Rösch, W., Moser, K. (Ed.). Stuttgart: Schattauer 1973

2.10

Blind Liver Needle Biopsy

G. MENGHINI

2.10.1 Instruments

Biopsy Needles. The needle is 7 cm long. Accessory arresting devices can limit the depth of penetration to 6, 5, or 4 cm respectively (Fig. 1). The wall of the needle is extremely thin (about 90 μm), and the tip has a characteristic bird's beak profile. A stylet inside the needle serves to prevent aspiration of the biopsy core into the syringe at the moment of tissue excision (Fig. 2).

The needle is available in four different sizes: 0.85 mm, 1.00 mm, 1.20 mm, and 1.40 mm internal diameter (ID). Needles of larger caliber, up to 2.00 mm, can be obtained for special indications, but these definitely should not be used in routine clinical practice [1–4].

Choice of Needle Size. The 1.20-mm diameter needle is recom-

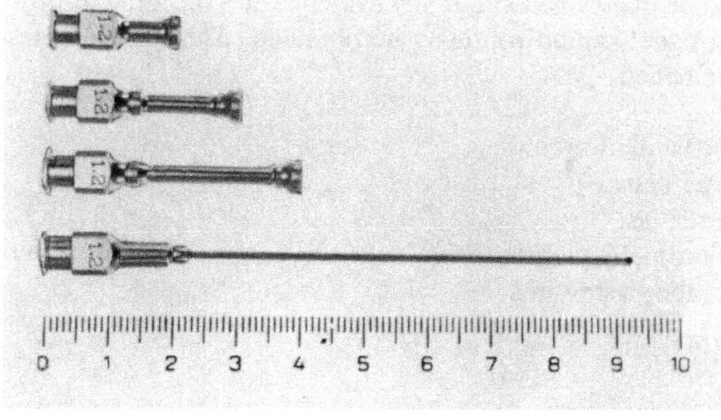

Fig. 1. A 1.2-mm needle with arresting devices of varying lengths.

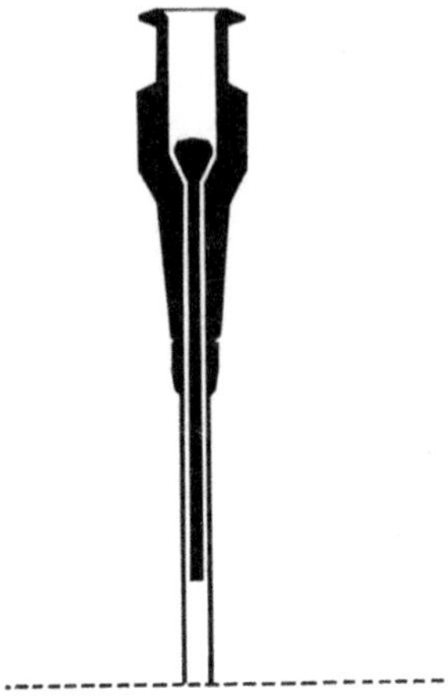

Fig. 2. Schematic longitudinal section through the biopsy needle.

mended for routine use. One of the arresting devices mentioned above may be attached to predetermine the depth to which the needle penetrates the liver (Fig. 1). The 1.40-mm needle may be used by experienced operators under special circumstances. The smaller calibers of 0.85 and 1.00 mm are reserved for high-risk situations, such as obstructive jaundice, acute passive congestion, tumors, etc. The 0.85-mm needle, which causes minimal trauma, is well suited for the diagnosis of neoplasia and certain diffuse hepatic diseases, including heavy metal and pigment storage disorders and steatosis.

2.10.2 Patient Preparation

The patient should be questioned about any evidence of a bleeding disorder, and a coagulation panel should routinely be obtained. The following tests are usually recommended:

1) Lee-White coagulation time
2) Bleeding time (Duke)
3) Rumpel-Leede test
4) Prothrombin time (Quick)
5) Partial thromboplastin time
6) Thrombocyte count
7) Clot retraction

No sedation is needed. It is advisable to perform the biopsy in the morning with the patient fasting for 12 h [4].

2.10.3 Postprocedure Care

After the biopsy, the patient is advised to lie on his right side for 2 h with the elbow pressing against the biopsy site. Pulse rate and blood pressure should be checked at 3-h intervals for the following 24 h.

2.10.4 Technique

Biopsy Site. We usually employ the intercostal approach. The site of skin puncture is determined simply by percussing the upper and lower margins of the liver [4] and is selected to coincide with the area of maximum dullness. The intercostal space actually selected is immaterial, but the needle should not be inserted anterior to the anterior axillary line.

The subcostal approach should be used only when the liver edge descends at least 3 cm below the costal margin; the liver should be palpable, both, during in- and expiration.

Patient Position. We biopsy with the patient supine and slightly turned to the left. The right arm is adducted so that the right hand grasps the edge of the bed to the left of the head [ref. 1–4].

Instrument Preparation. About 2 ml of isotonic saline are aspirated into a 5-cc tight-fitting syringe. The syringe is attached to the biopsy needle, and the patency of the needle is checked by expelling about one-half of the saline.

The isotonic solution serves the following purposes: (a) to clear skin fragments and subcutaneous tissues from the needle that might otherwise decrease the chances of obtaining an adequate tissue cylinder and (b) to facilitate expulsion of the liver core at the end of the procedure [1].

Anesthesia. Skin and the full thickness of the intercostal space are infiltrated with a fine (No. 22 or 24), short (2.0 cm) needle. The direction should be that of the path to be taken by the biopsy needle. Two to three milliliters of a local anesthetic (Novocain or lidocaine) usually suffice.

Apnea Training. The patient should remain apneic for 4–5 s during the intrahepatic phase of the biopsy procedure. Apnea in deep expiration, as used earlier, is not necessary; rather, it is sufficient to hold the breath at the end of normal expiration [4]. It is advisable to practice this with the patient after local anesthesia has been administered, to avoid delays and misunderstandings during the biopsy itself. The physician watches the patient breathe and orders him to stop at the end of a normal expiration. This is repeated until the patient complies with the order promptly.

Skin Perforation. We prefer to penetrate the skin with a suitable trocar to a depth of 2–3 mm at the site chosen for biopsy (Fig. 3). The biopsy needle can then be advanced into the subcutaneous tissue without encountering resistance at the skin surface.

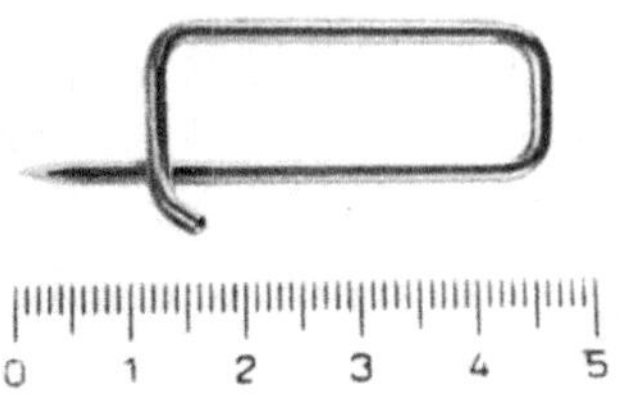

Fig. 3. Trocar for skin perforation.

2.10.4.1 Slow (Extrahepatic) Phase

2.10.4.1.1 Penetration into Subcutaneous Tissue (Fig. 5/1). Using the previously placed skin incision, the needle is advanced until the subcutaneous tissue is reached. The depth of penetration should not exceed 3–4 mm.

2.10.4.1.2 Clearing of Tissue Particles (Fig. 5/2). One-half of the syringe contents are injected, thereby expelling remnants of skin and fatty tissue that may have entered the needle. The remaining one-half of the saline should stay in the syringe.

2.10.4.1.3 Apneic Phase. At this point, the patient should hold his breath. The same words and intonation should be used as during the prior practice session.

2.10.4.1.4 Needle Position and Aspiration (Fig. 5/3). The needle should be held at right angles to the skin surface with slight posterior deviation. Next, a strong vacuum is created by pulling the plunger back as far as possible. Correct position of the physician's hands is of critical importance: An error may cause the procedure to be unsuccessful. The head of the plunger is grasped between the right thumb and middle finger. It is then retracted to its limit and fixed in this position by the extended index finger, which rests against the syringe sleeve. This position must be maintained during the following maneuver. The left middle finger and thumb hold the needle hub; the left index finger rests transversely against the arresting sleeve (Fig. 4).

2.10.4.2 Rapid (Intrahepatic) Phase

2.10.4.2.1 Needle Introduction into the Liver (Fig. 5/4). With the syringe under maximal aspiration, the needle is pushed straight into the liver without torsion or lateral deviation.

2.10.4.2.2 Needle Extraction (Fig. 5/5). As soon as maximum penetration has been achieved, the needle is suddenly pulled out in the same direction as during its introduction. Again, the motion should be completely

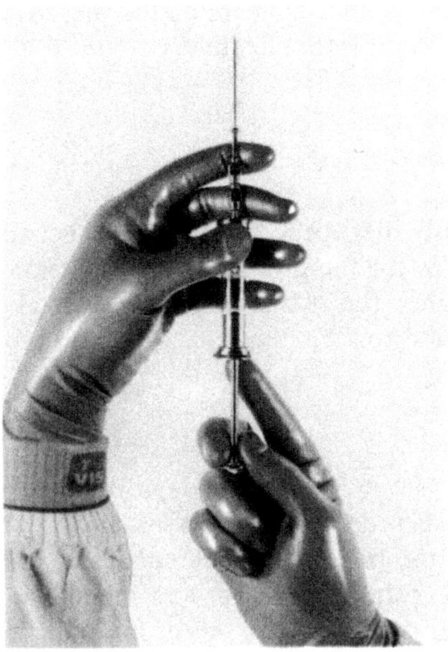

Fig. 4. Position of hands and fingers during the intrahepatic phase.

straight, without rotation or lateral movement. The syringe remains in aspiration to avoid loss of the tissue core after removal of the needle. The procedure is now completed. The swift motions during the intrahepatic phase should be accomplished in less than 1 s [1,6].

Expulsion of the Biopsy Core. The tip of the biopsy needle is simply submerged into a small beaker or cup containing a few milliliters of normal saline. The suction on the syringe is released slowly and, finally, all

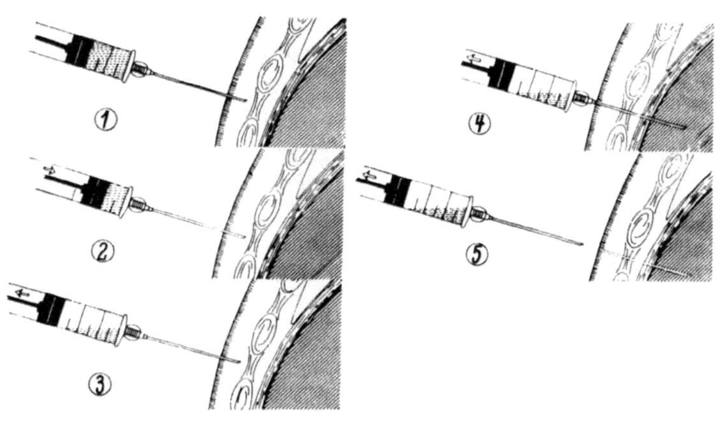

Fig. 5. Schematic illustration of the different phases of aspiration liver biopsy.

syringe contents are expelled. The tissue cylinder appears and is placed on a piece of filter or lens paper before placing it into a fixative.

2.10.5 Indications

Liver needle biopsy is helpful and usually diagnostic for all diffuse hepatic diseases. It may also give important clues for the presence of focal lesions. The method can be applied routinely since the risk is negligible, provided the guidelines described above are adhered to.

2.10.6 Contraindications

Absolute contraindications include all disorders of hemostasis and infections of pleura, peritoneum, liver, and the bile ducts. Echinococcus cysts may cause severe complications, including shock. Another contraindication is the absence of liver dullness to percussion. However, repeat examination will frequently reveal initially unrecognized liver dullness, allowing the procedure to be carried out.

Relative contraindications include obstructive jaundice, ascites, fever, and cachexia. The rapid method of liver biopsy has greatly decreased the number of contraindications that existed with the older techniques. The remaining contraindications, however, must be strictly observed.

2.10.7 Complications

While serious complications are extremely rare, they may occur, and the physician should be aware of this possibility. Some patients complain of right shoulder pain, beginning either immediately after the biopsy, or 1–2 h later. The pain usually is not severe and does not require specific intervention. Its incidence lies between 5% and 10%. Serious complications are bile peritonitis, pleural and peritoneal bleeding, and pneumothorax. With few exceptions, these can be ascribed to technical errors or to incorrect patient selection.

References

1. MENGHINI, G.: One second needle biopsy of the liver. Gastroenterology *35*, 190–199 (1958)
2. MENGHINI, G.: Two-operator needle biopsy of the liver. Am. J. Dig. Dis. *4*, 682–692 (1959)

3. Menghini, G.: Probleme der Leberbiopsie. In: Fortschritte der Gastroenterologie. Wildhirt, E. (ed.), S. 222–230. München, Berlin: Urban & Schwarzenberg 1960
4. Menghini, G.: One second biopsy of the liver. Problems of its clinical application. N. Engl. J. Med. *283*, 582–585 (1970)
5. Lindner, H.: Das Risiko der perkutanen Leberbiopsie. Med. Klin. *66*, 924–929 (1971)
6. Thaler, H.: Leberbiopsie. Berlin, Heidelberg, New York: Springer 1969

2.11
Laparoscopy

H. LINDNER/P. FRÜHMORGEN

Laparoscopy is a low-risk method of high diagnostic efficacy. Thorough familiarity with gentle performance of this technique is an absolute prerequisite. This knowledge should be acquired at an institution where a large number of examinations are carried out, reinforced by audiovisual methods, e.g., instructional movies [12,14], and extended by the study of textbooks and atlases [1,13].

The procedure can be performed in a darkened endoscopy suite or in an operating room. The basic equipment is listed in Table 1. Laparoscopy is an aseptic examination of the peritoneal cavity; it is not a mini-laparotomy. The need for sterile precautions outside the peritoneum extends only to maintaining asepsis of the instruments which are to be introduced. No infectious complications have been observed under these conditions. The endoscopy nurse, wearing sterile gloves, arranges the required instruments on two or three movable tables (Table 2).

Table 1. Basic equipment for laparoscopy.

Freely movable endoscopy table (the Maquet endoscopy table, No. 1531.90 is recommended)
Light source of 250 W capacity and electronic flash generator for distal electronic flash photography
1 metal-covered light cable (autoclavable to 120° C)
Camera
Riwo objectives of 95, 110, and 135 mm focal length (should be purchased in this order)
Insufflation apparatus: N_2O pneu-automatic
Water gun for cleaning
High-frequency diathermy unit with accessories (Martin Elektrotom 120 or Erbe R 3)
Polaroid camera

Table 2. Laparoscopy instrumentation.

I.

- Local anesthesia
  - 10-ml disposable syringe
  - Small-caliber needle for intracutaneous injection
  - Larger needle, 10 cm long
  - Container with 50 ml 1% mepivacaine HCl
- Pneumoperitoeneum
  - Veress needle with Luer-Lok connector
  - 50-ml syringe for determining needle position (aspiration and trial insufflation)
- Disposable scalpel
- Laparoscope trocar with cannula (10-mm diameter)
- Instruments for liver biopsy (Menghini or Vim-Silverman)
- Probe for electrocoagulation
- Wound closure
  - Forceps
  - Needle holder
  - Needle
  - Cotton suture material, size 0, or
  - Sterile strip
- Cotton swab
- Container with 10 ml of physiologic saline

II.

- Laparoscopes (in sequence of purchase), prewarmed by heating pad in sterile towel or in heating apparatus with autoclavable tubes
  - Lumina laparoscope, 130° view deflection, 10-mm diameter
    - Optics for photolaparoscope, 130° view deflection; distal electronic flash tube
    - Lumina operating laparoscope, 170° view deflection (Fig. 2)
    - Vario-photolaparoscope optics, 130° view deflection; equipped for viewing with electronic flash carrier and distal flash tube

III.

- Light cable
- Insufflation conduit with Luer-Lok connector (for use with the N_2O insufflation apparatus of Siede)
- Cable for coagulation electrode
- Metal stethoscope (autoclavable)
- Forceps, scissors, needle holder, needles, small curved clamps (back-up)
- Reserve rubber gaskets
- Freiburg set for second access to the abdomen; set with a longer cannula may also be used for the operating laparoscope (Fig. 2)
  - Biopsy forceps
  - Operating laparoscope
  - Trocar with cannula
    - Biopsy forceps
    - Curved scissors
    - Blunt grasping forceps
    - Double-cupped forceps
    - Biopsy forceps with lancette-type jaws (Robbers forceps)
    - Coagulation electrode
    - Menghini biopsy needle
    - Knife
    - Graduated measuring probe

2.11.1 Instruments

2.11.1.1 Optical Instruments

Several instruments are commercially available. We prefer the Lumina laparoscopes (Wolf, Knittlinger) because our experience has shown these to be superior to other optical systems, particularly for photography [10,11]. The new Lumina laparoscope with variable optics is equipped with an eyepiece that can be adjusted for inspection of whole organs as well as for evaluation of fine structural details without changing position of the instrument tip [7].

Complications due to the 10-mm size of the standard trocar have not been observed. The small caliber Menghini laparoscope with Lumina optics is useful for cases in which the differential diagnosis of ascites is the main objective and the presence of decompensated portal hypertension cannot be ruled out preoperatively. The trocar of this instrument is only 6 mm in diameter, which decreases the risk of an ascitic fluid leak.

The laparoscope is equipped with a wide-angle objective that has an optical field of about 60° to provide a panoramic view despite the short viewing distance available. In 1942, H. Kalk proposed incorporation of a viewing angle of 130°. The advantage of this classic viewing angle of 50° (or 130°) is that it directs the central light beam at a 90° angle to the liver surface in the presence of normal topographic conditions. With forward-viewing optics of 27.5° or 152.5°, and even more with optics of 170° and 180°, the liver is seen tangentially and surface variations are difficult to assess. The magnification factor of the Lumina laparoscope (Fig. 1) is ×6.1 at 1 cm distance, ×2 at 3 cm, and ×1 at 6 cm. The object appears smaller than natural size at distances greater than 6 cm. This allows the operator a view of much of the intraperitoneal surfaces during withdrawal of the instrument.

2.11.1.2 Accessory Instruments

A number of accessory instruments can be introduced through the Lumina operating laparoscope (Fig. 2) or through a second penetration with an additional trocar (biopsy set, model Freiburg) which usually is placed in the right upper quadrant [1]. Although this requires a second area of local anesthesia, the additional penetration permits easier and safer manipulation of instruments within the abdomen than working with the operating laparoscope alone. A second access to the peritoneal cavity is always required for transhepatic cholangiography under laparoscopic control, which we perform with the Chiba needle. A graduated probe is used to palpate gallbladder and liver, to lift up both hepatic lobes for examination of the posterior surface, and to probe suspicious structures within the abdomen. The size of organs and lesions can thus be determined directly.

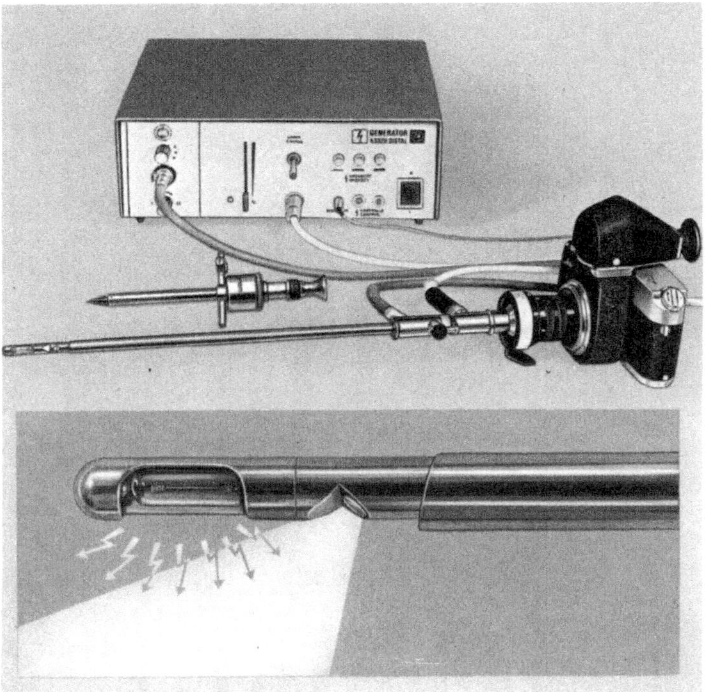

Fig. 1. Photolaparoscope with 130° deflection of view and combined light source. Distal end with intra-abdominal electronic flash (Richard Wolf GmbH, Knittlingen).

2.11.2 Patient Preparation

2.11.2.1 Initial Examination

a) The general clinical evaluation should be completed, leading to specific questions to be answered by the laparoscopist.
b) Coagulation defects must be excluded. A prothrombin time of 40% and a platelet count of 40,000 constitute the lower permissible limit. The partial thromboplastin time should be normal.
c) Routine electrocardiogram.
d) Chest radiograph.

2.11.2.2 Preparation of the Patient

a) Patient reassurance by explaining the procedure and by obtaining informed consent; this should be done by the physician.

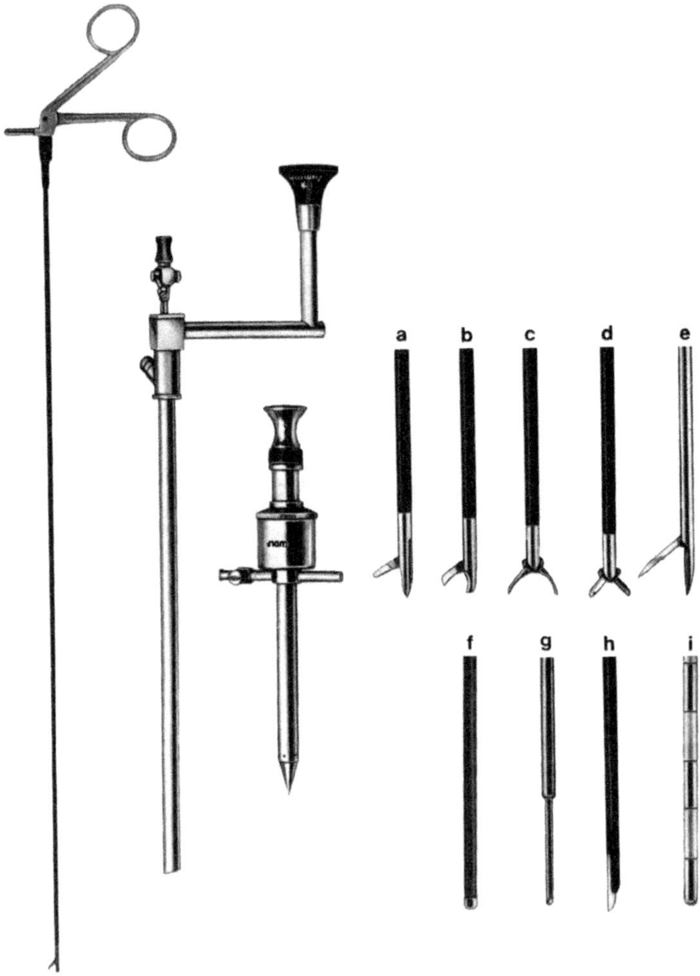

Fig. 2. Lumina operating laparoscope with accessory instruments; these may also be used with the Freiburg set (see Table 2/III).

b) Inguinal, femoral, and incisional hernias are taped tightly. Hiatus hernia is not a contraindication.
c) Light supper and sedative at bedtime, if needed.
d) The patient should urinate and defecate before the procedure; he should be fasting since midnight.
e) Shaving and mechanical cleansing of the abdominal wall.
f) Prophylactic antibiotics are not indicated.
g) Triflupromazine, 20 mg IM, 2 h before the procedure.

h) A mixture of oxycodone HCl, 10 mg, plus scopolamine HBr, 0.5 mg, plus ephedrine HCl, 25 mg, SC, 1 h before the procedure (for patients up to 65 years).

In the presence of high-grade (obstructive) jaundice and with elderly patients, we prefer, instead, to give meperidine HCl, 50–100 mg IV, after the pneumoperitoneum needle is introduced.

Alternatively: diazepam, 20–80 mg and meperidine HCl IV in doses adjusted to body weight.

The medication dosage needs to be individualized and additional dose increments may have to be given during the examination. Diazepam has the advantage of inducing retrograde amnesia. Venous thromboses should be prevented by using a large antecubital vein which is kept open by a saline drip. A large-bore needle should be employed to facilitate rapid volume substitution should vascular collapse occur.

i) Restless patients receive additional diazepam intravenously, which may, however, have a paradoxical effect. The procedure becomes needlessly difficult when the patient has received insufficient sedative and analgesic medication.

j) Successful medical therapy of ascites. Large volumes of ascitic fluid should only be removed when it is caused by peritoneal carcinomatosis or tuberculosis. Hepatic coma may be precipitated by paracentesis when the ascites is due to liver disease.

2.11.3 Postprocedure Care

Pulse rate should be charted on a flow sheet every 15 min and blood pressure every 30 min for 3 h. Hourly vital signs are obtained for the next 6 h. The dressing should be inspected after 15 min for unusual bleeding. The patient should lie supine; the head need not be lowered. Discharge may be arranged for the 1st or 2nd postoperative day, unless further hospitalization is required for other reasons. The patient usually is totally asymptomatic within 24 h, provided the procedure was carried out gently and by competent hands.

2.11.4 Technique

For routine laparoscopy, only one endoscopy nurse is needed to monitor the patient, help with photography, and, wearing sterile gloves, hand the instruments to the physician. More assistants are needed with high-risk laparoscopies, with combined radiologic-endoscopic examinations, and for teaching purposes.

The abdominal skin is prepared as for a laparotomy, from three fingerbreadths above the symphysis to three to four fingerbreadths below the nipples. The patient is covered with clean towels, leaving free a large quadratic area of the abdomen. The examiner wears a clean gown and sterile, disposable gloves. The indifferent electrode for coagulation with the high-frequency diathermy unit is attached to the patient as he is placed on the table.

2.11.4.1 Pneumoperitoneum

The border between the lateral and the middle third of the Richter-Monroe line (Fig. 3) is marked for introduction of the Veress needle, and local anesthesia is given with no more than 10 ml of 1% mepivacaine HCl. This point is selected because there is no danger of injury to large vessels such as aorta, vena cava, and common iliac artery by the pneumoperitoneum needle, with possible air embolism. The contralateral side is used when postappendectomy adhesions may be present. Following skin puncture with a disposable scalpel, the Veress needle is introduced by holding the ridged part without blocking the Luer-Lok connector (Fig. 4). The patient is asked to bear down and let the abdominal wall protrude. The characteristic resistance by fascia and peritoneum are easily appreciated as the needle is advanced. The blunt stylet protrudes spontaneously from the sharp cannula as soon as tissue resistance ceases and the peritoneum has been entered.

With adipose patients, the Veress needle may have to be introduced at the site selected for the laparoscopy trocar since penetration of the fascia is more easily noticed there than in the thick layers of adipose tissue of the lower abdomen. Use of this site also avoids foam formation in the presence of ascites. Some examiners select this site routinely [5]. It is im-

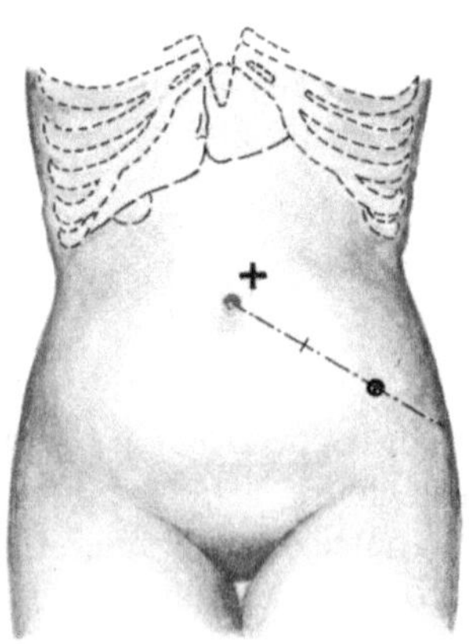

Fig. 3. Richter-Monroe line with point of introduction of the Veress needle and the classic site of insertion of the laparoscope trocar.

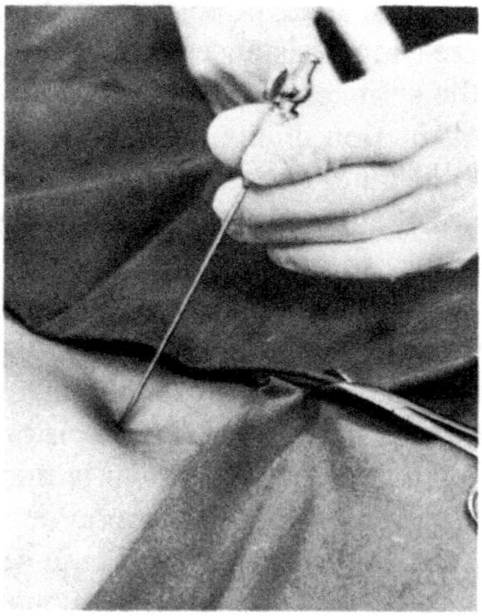

Fig. 4. Veress needle during introduction.

perative that the free position of the cannula be verified: Neither blood nor intestinal contents should appear upon aspiration with a 50-ml syringe; 20 cm^3 of air should be insufflated without encountering resistance and without being able to be reaspirated.

The N_2O pneu unit is connected at this point. It automatically records gas flow and pressure. N_2O is tolerated without complications and is resorbed nearly as fast as CO_2. CO_2 is not suitable for routine laparoscopy since it irritates the peritoneum, causing local vasodilatation and pain.

Air insufflation with a 100-ml syringe and a two-way stopcock is no longer acceptable since it requires additional personnel, adds to the duration of the procedure, and causes increased patient discomfort due to the slow resorption of N_2 from the peritoneum.

Free gas flow into the peritoneal cavity produces a continuous rushing sound that can be heard with a sterile stethoscope held over the tip of the needle. Liver dullness disappears after insufflation of 300–500 cm^3 of N_2O. The usual volume needed in adults is 2 liters, with a maximum of 5 liters.

The pneumoperitoneum develops automatically under constant observation of the N_2O pneu unit: filling pressure of 10–18 mm Hg with resistance by the Veress needle of less than 8 mm Hg; the sphere of the gas flow indicator is located at the upper end of the glass cylinder.

2.11.4.2 Introduction of the Laparoscope

In the meantime, the examiner applies local anesthesia for the laparoscope trocar with 20–40 ml of 1% mepivacaine HCl. Intracutaneous injection is followed by infiltration of subcutaneous tissue and abdominal muscle and, finally, by thorough preperitoneal anesthesia. Inadvertent penetration of the peritoneum is signaled by pain, decreasing resistance to injection, and by the ability to aspirate N_2O gas into the syringe.

The conventional puncture site for introduction of the laparoscope is two fingerbreadths above the umbilicus and not quite two fingerbreadths to the left of the midline, at the medial border of the rectus abdominis muscle (Fig. 5). Puncture further to the left risks injury to the superior epigastric artery; puncture to the right of the umbilicus might penetrate the ligamentum teres with damage to a paraumbilical or a persisting umbilical vein.

The success of the entire procedure often depends on the intelligent choice of the point where the laparoscope trocar is introduced. The decision should always be based on careful palpation of anatomic landmarks and on anticipated adhesions as the result of prior abdominal operations. The overriding concern should be to choose conditions that allow adequate visualization of the organ in question—usually the liver. The conventional puncture site described above may have to be varied with these considerations in mind. When the liver is very large, or when midline adhesions are to be expected as a result of gastric resection, a point to the left and below the umbilicus may be preferred. Even the umbilicus is not a constant landmark since it is displaced caudally in very obese patients and those with ascites.

The examiner confirms the presence of a gas-fluid level by aspirating gas and by needle palpation. A sufficiently large pneumoperitoneum is required for the safe and diagnostically effective performance of the procedure.

The trocar, with its relatively atraumatic conical tip, is first directed parallel to the belt line for about 1 cm and then advanced through the abdominal wall with a rotating motion (Fig. 5). The patient is asked to bear down. The trocar is withdrawn as soon as trocar and cannula have entered the peritoneal cavity; the valve closes automatically.

The use of modern fiberoptic laparoscopes makes it possible to work in a dimly lit rather than a dark room. Thus, the physician is better able to observe the entire situation, and the endoscopy nurse can monitor the patient more closely.

Less experienced physicians initially prefer a forward-viewing laparoscope, such as the operating laparoscope, because one can already see from within the trocar cannula whether the abdomen has been entered and because orientation appears easier initially. However, this instrument should never be used for diagnostic purposes.

If a mother-of-pearl-like tissue plane is seen, the hollow trocar cannula is still located preperitoneally. The trocar should then be reinserted and advanced further, together with the cannula.

No condensation will form on the instrument in the peritoneal cavity, provided the laparoscope has been prewarmed to about 50° C. Vision is im-

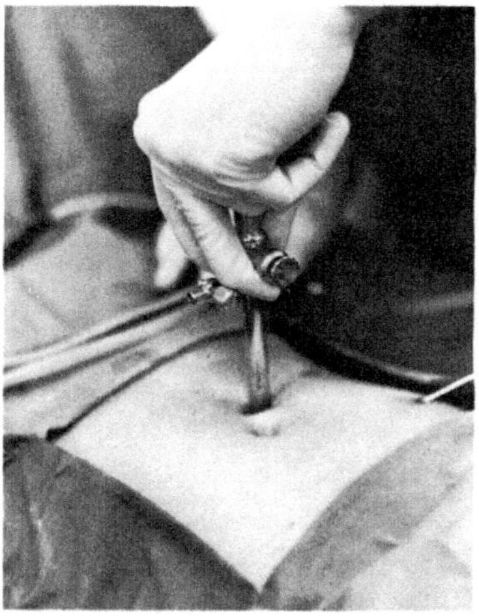

Fig. 5. Introduction of the laparoscope trocar.

paired when the optical system is smudged by blood, fat, or ascites present in the trocar or abdomen. The only remedy consists of careful cleaning with warm, sterile physiologic saline.

The view may be obstructed by adhesions. These may be cut with curved forceps introduced through the operating laparoscope, unless they are vascular or very dense. Most adhesions, however, can be pushed aside as the laparoscope is advanced.

Lysis of adhesions by endothermia has recently proved quite successful in our hands. The tissue is heated to 80° C, which causes the blood vessels to thrombose, preventing bleeding after the adhesions are severed. This procedure is of therapeutic benefit in the Fitz-Hugh–Curtis syndrome, characterized by painful adhesions as a consequence of intraperitoneal gonorrhea.

Occasionally, gas is insufflated dorsal to the greater omentum, causing it and the transverse colon to rise to the ventral aspect of the peritoneum. Thus, the liver is obscured and only loops of small bowel can be seen. When this characteristic picture is encountered, the trocar cannula has to be withdrawn. Percussion of the abdominal wall causes the omentum to fall back into its usual position and the liver becomes visible.

2.11.4.3 Inspection

The free position of the Veress needle is confirmed first. When its tip is seen to have entered the omentum, the organ is freed by a rocking motion. Inexperienced hands may cause omental emphysema. Additional N_2O may be insufflated through the torcar when gas-containing omentum interferes with adequate inspection.

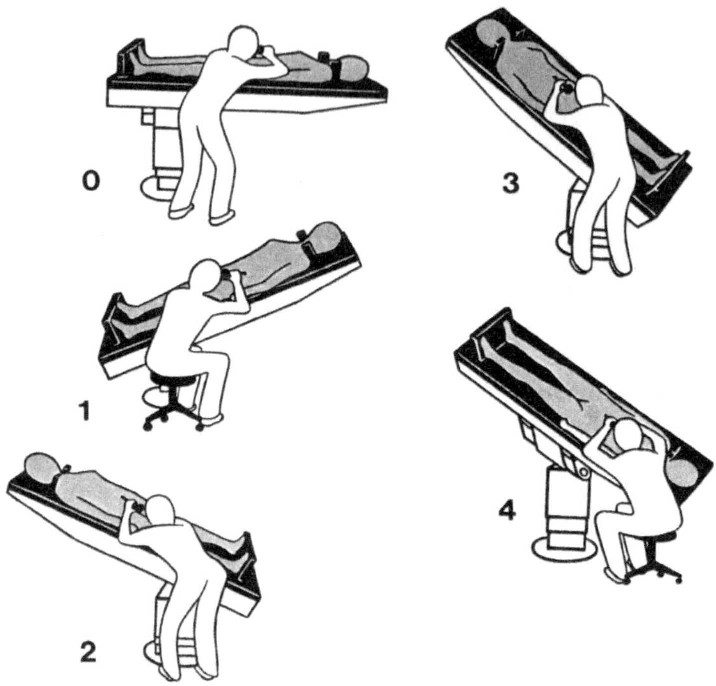

Fig. 6. Typical position for inspection of the entire accessible peritoneal space.

The movable Maquet examining table (Fig. 6), driven by an electric motor, facilitates changing the patient's position. This permits inspection of the entire peritoneal cavity by following a defined sequence of maneuvers (Table 3; Fig. 6). Important information, particularly second lesions, are overlooked all too frequently unless a certain routine is adhered to.

The endoscopist should watch the patient very closely during examination in position 3, which may lead to hypotension and collapse. The patient is advised to report developing dizzyness, nausea, and dyspnea. These complaints disappear soon after the head is lowered.

2.11.4.4 Biopsy

We prefer the Vim-Silverman needle in the presence of suspected chronic hepatitis and cirrhosis since it yields a large tissue cylinder which permits histologic estimation of the degree of fibrosis and pseudolobule formation. The Menghini needle is used in all other situations.

The Vim-Silverman needle is introduced either by direct percutaneous puncture or, tangientially, via the Freiburg set. The tip should penetrate

Table 3. Positions during laparoscopy (Fig. 6).

Position of examiner and endoscopy table	*Inspection with intraperitoneal panoramic view*
Position 0	
Examiner to the left of the patient; patient supine	Free position of Veress needle. Overview of entire abdomen and inspection of peritoneum. Search for injury by the trocar tip (blood!). Cecum, colon
Position 1	
Examiner to the left of the patient. Patient 15°–20° head-up; left lateral decubitus	Right (and left) hepatic lobe. Overview and inspection with magnification; falciform ligament and ligamentum teres. Standard position for liver biopsy.
Up to 45° head-up position and rotation	Lateral portion of right hepatic lobe
Position 2	
Examiner to the right of the patient. Patient 15°–20° head-up; right lateral decubitus	Left hepatic lobe, anterior and posterior aspects. Falciform ligament and ligamentum teres; minor omentum; pancreas, spleen; stomach up to cardia
Position 3	
Examiner to the right of the patient. Position 2 continued up to 45° head elevation (extreme position; only needed for short periods)	Spleen; phrenicocolic ligament; left triangular ligament; diaphragm with esophageal hiatus; esophagus
Position 4	
Examiner to the left of the patient; 40° head-down position; rotation to the left side by up to 45°	Cecum, appendix, peritoneum. True pelvis; adnexae and uterus

into the right hepatic lobe, lateral to the gallbladder, to a depth of about 1 cm. This site is easily seen through the laparoscope and is near the dome of the right lobe or just lateral to it. The stylet is removed, the two-pronged biopsy needle pushed in, and needle with cannula are advanced by a rotating motion. Major bleeding is rare with this technique because the biopsy is obtained from deep within the liver. Sufficient tissue is nearly always retrieved with the first attempt.

The less traumatic biopsy with the Menghini needle can be carried out through a separate puncture or through an operating laparoscope. With

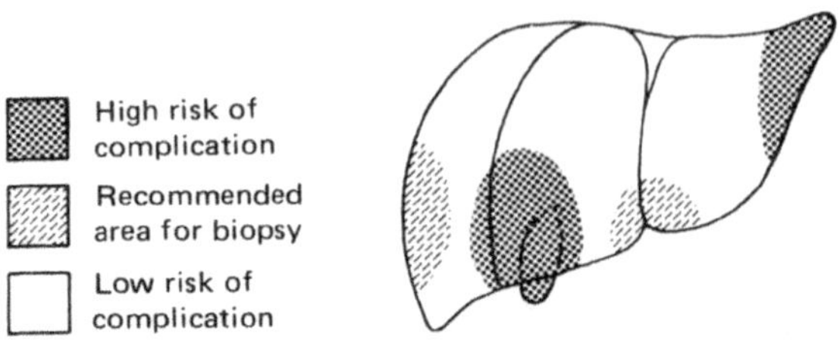

Fig. 7. Topography during liver biopsy.

either approach, the biopsy site should be well within view of the laparoscope; the area around the gallbladder should be avoided (Fig. 7). We prefer routinely the medial part of the right hepatic lobe. The left lobe should only be biopsied for circumscribed lesions or when both lobes differ in appearance. Its small anterior-posterior diameter may lead to penetration of the dorsal capsule by the needle with the resultant risk of undetected post-biopsy bleeding. The lateral aspect of the left lobe should never be biopsied; it is very thin and the danger of bleeding is accordingly high.

Circumscribed lesions of the liver surface, such as nodules and areas suspicious for carcinoma, can safely be excised with the Robbers forceps. When hypervascularization is noted with its increased risk of bleeding, we prefer to carry out a thin needle biopsy with either the Menghini or Chiba model.

Most postbiopsy bleeding stops spontaneously. If not, a thermocautery button probe is introduced through the cannula of the Vim-Silverman needle, through the operating laparoscope, or the channel used for accessory instruments. The tract made by the biopsy needle in the liver is then electrocoagulated. Alternative methods for hemostasis are simple compression with a probe, reintroduction of the Vim-Silverman needle with stylet into the biopsy tract, and injection of epinephrine or thrombin solution into and on the biopsy track.

Bleeding that does not respond to the above measures may be stopped by compression with a cotton swab soaked with thrombin solution; the swab is manipulated through the operating laparoscope with a grasping forceps. Finally, a suitably trimmed piece of Gelfoam or fibrin foam may be applied in the same fashion.

When splenomegaly without portal hypertension is the presenting diagnostic problem, splenic biopsy can be carried out with the Menghini needle without significant risk.

2.11.4.5 Combined Radiologic-Endoscopic Examination

Combination of radiologic methods with laparoscopy offers further diagnostic possibilities that will not be discussed in this brief overview [16].

2.11.4.6 Laparoscopic Photography

Laparoscopy without photographic documentation is analogous to the antiquated practice of thorax fluoroscopy without a radiographic chest film. The purpose of laparoscopy lies not only in obtaining liver biopsies under direct observation. All findings should be documented and evaluated according to objective criteria. The photographic picture is the objective document of macroscopic changes and may reveal important additional findings that were not realized during the procedure itself.

Negative color film is used for routine photography; 5 × 5 cm positive prints are attached to the patient's chart and filed for research purposes; 35-mm transparencies are prepared for presentation at meetings. The Polaroid camera is used in situations where photographic documentation has to be available immediately.

The intra-abdominal electronic flash has been claimed to cause extrasystoles. This statement, however, is contradicted by theoretical considerations, experimental results, and by practical experience. The distal electronic flash is, in fact, very safe. All electric connections and the cover over the flash unit should, of course, be checked to avoid entry of moisture. Otherwise, the flash unit will not work.

The results obtained with color photography using an intra-abdominal flash are far superior to those obtained with an extracorporeal flash. This has been demonstrated convincingly by our comparative investigations [10,11]. When carrying out photography, it must be remembered that only those areas will be reproduced well on the film that were clear to the examiner's eye. Satisfactory results will be obtained by photographing in the focal plane, avoiding too strong a tangential illumination, and using a flash intensity matched to the "brightness" of the organ and its distance from the objective, or else by selecting objectives of various focal lengths, between 70 and 110 mm. The brightness is markedly influenced by the color of the liver. A yellow "fatty" liver will reflect the light to a considerably greater degree than will the dark-green liver found in obstructive jaundice.

2.11.5 Indications

1) Differential diagnosis of jaundice
2) Explanation for abnormally elevated serum enzymes
3) Explanation for hepato- and splenomegaly
    a) Chronic hepatitis
    b) Cirrhosis with or without portal hypertension
    c) Hepatic fibrosis
    d) Hepatic cysts
    e) Echinococcal disease

4) Ascites of unknown etiology
5) Laparoscopic exploration
   a) Suspected malignancy
   b) Rule out metastases with known primary tumor
   c) Chronic abdominal symptoms
   d) Adhesions, chronic appendicitis, adnexitis
   e) Differential diagnosis of inflammatory and neoplastic diseases of the gallbladder (nonvisualization on oral cholecystogram)
6) Emergency laparoscopy
7) Gynecologic diagnostic problems

In Germany, the predominating role of laparoscopy in the morphologic diagnosis of liver diseases is accepted. The German medical community realizes the limitations of the exclusive use of blind percutaneous liver biopsy, which yields false negative or misleading diagnostic information in 20%–50% of cases with chronic hepatitis and cirrhosis.

The dilemma of a histologic diagnosis without macroscopic observation represents a frequent indication for laparoscopy in view of the sampling error of the blind biopsy. Laparoscopy is needed when the liver appears indurated on palpation, particularly when there is any discrepancy between clinical observation and the result of the percutaneous biopsy. The role of the latter procedure is primarily to provide serial observations of diffuse hepatic diseases, which were originally diagnosed by laparoscopy [9].

Laparoscopy should also be performed in each instance of diagnostically unresolved nonvisualization on oral cholecystography, especially when carcinoma of the gallbladder has to be considered, as well as to convince the occasional patient of the need for gallbladder surgery. With routine inspection of all accessible abdominal organs, preoperative laparoscopy is finding increased application to determine operability of malignant tumors and to avoid unnecessary surgical procedures. In many cases, laparoscopy can replace exploratory laparotomy, especially for staging of lymphomas, including Hodgkin's disease. The capabilities of emergency laparoscopy are still largely unappreciated [4].

2.11.6 Contraindications

Laparoscopy should be avoided, if possible, in the presence of decompensated cirrhosis with portal hypertension and ascites. Indications should be applied conservatively to patients with coronary artery disease since a few instances of myocardial infarction have occurred during the procedure. Absolute contraindications are severe bleeding disorders, advanced cor pulmonale, congestive heart failure in general, and severe arterial hypertension. In contrast to past opinions, hiatus hernia does not represent a contraindication [5].

2.11.7 Complications

1) Preperitoneal and omental emphysema
2) Bleeding from the site of penetration of the abdominal wall, especially injury to large vessels by the Veress needle with resulting severe hemorrhage or air embolism
3) Injury by the laparoscope trocar with perforation of adherent intestinal loops, penetration of the liver capsule, or rupture of large vessels, especially with portal hypertension (caput Medusae!)
4) Tearing of adhesions with bleeding
5) Mediastinal emphysema
6) Shock with cardiac arrhythmias
7) Complications of liver biopsy (see Sect. 2.11.4.4)

According to Brühl, the combined experience of many centers revealed a mortality of 0.29% with 63,845 laparoscopies, which included 48,766 liver biopsies [2]. The leading causes of death were bile peritonitis (eight cases) and bleeding (seven cases). A more recent statistic by Look in 1974 showed an even lower mortality rate of 0.014%.

The risk of any operative diagnostic method is not completely represented by mortality figures. Table 4, therefore, lists the incidence of nonfatal complications.

Table 4. Complications during 63,845 laparoscopies that included 48,766 liver biopsies under direct vision.

Bleeding	42
Bile peritonitis	34
Cutaneous emphysema	366
Omental emphysema	803
Mediastinal emphysema	50
Intestinal perforation	47
Pneumothorax	18
Air embolism	1
Hernias	8
Severe shock	166
Miscellaneous	40
Deaths	19
Total	1594

References

1. BECK, K.: Atlas der Laparoskopie. Stuttgart: Schattauer 1968
2. BRÜHL, W.: Zwischenfälle und Komplikationen bei der Laparoskopie und gezielter Leberpunktion. Dtsch. Med. Wochenschr. *91*, 2297 (1966)
3. ERB, W., KRÖHL, R.: Über die Füllung des Pneumoperitoneums mit verschiedenen Gasen. In: Grundlagen und Fortschritte der Laparoskopie. LINDNER, H. (Ed.). Gräfelfing: Demeter 1970
4. FAHRLÄNDER, H.: Die Laparoskopie bei abdominellen Notfällen. Dtsch. Med. Wochenschr. *94*, 890 (1969)
5. HENNING, H.: Die Laparoskopie bei der Hiatushernie. In: Grundlagen und Fortschritte der Laparoskopie. LINDNER, H., (Ed.). Gräfelfing: Demeter 1970
6. HENNING, H., LOOK, D., v. BRAUN, H., LÜDERS, C. J.: Die Laparoskopie heute. Internist. Prax. *11*, 385 (1972) and *12* (31), 385 (1972)
7. LENT, H.: Versuche zu einer Vario-Optik. In: Fortschritte der gastroenterologischen Endoskopie. LINDNER, H. (Ed.). Vol. V. Baden-Baden: Witzstrock 1973
8. LINDNER, H.: Die perkutane Leberbiopsie mit der Menghininadel. Med. Welt 2265 (1962)
9. LINDNER, H.: Grenzen und Gefahren der perkutanen Leberbiopsie mit der Menghininadel. Dtsch. Med. Wochenschr. *92*, 1751 (1967)
10. LINDNER, H.: Endoscopy *1*, 1 (1969)
11. LINDNER, H.: Die zwei Prinzipien der laparoskopischen Technik: Panoramaübersicht und Lupenbetrachtung. In: Moderne gastroenterologische Endoskopie. HEINKEL, K., LINDNER, H. (Ed.). Gräfelfing: Demeter 1971
12. LINDNER, H.: The technique of laparoscopy. 16 mm Farbtonfilm im Verleth Dr. Madaus Köln 1972
13. LINDNER, H. (ed.): Laparoskopie und Leberbiopsie. New York: Witzstrock, 1975
14. LINDNER, H.: Indications for Laparoscopy 16 mm color movie with audio. On loan from Dr. Madaus Köln 1977
15. VIDO, E., WINCKLER, K.: Diagnose der Leberzirrhose anhand laparoskopischer und histologischer Befunde. Med. Klin. *67*, 400 (1972)
16. WANNAGAT, L.: Indikation zur direkten Cholecystcholangiographie und Cholangiographie. Dtsch. Med. Wochenschr. *94*, 2111 (1969)
17. WILDHIRT, E.: Bedeutung und Wert der Laparoskopie und gezielten Leberpunktion. Stuttgart: Thieme: 1964
18. WILDHIRT, E.: Laparoskopie und Leberbiopsie. Wien. Med. Wochenschr. *120*, 66 (1970)

2.12

Laparoscopic Inspection and Biopsy of the Pancreas

D. LOOK/H. HENNING

2.12.1 Instruments

Instrumentation cannula (3-mm diameter) with trocar and automatic valve, palpation probe, scissors, and biopsy forceps with two cupped jaws taken from the accessories of the operating laparoscope of Jacobs-Palmer. Injection needle, 20-cm long, 0,9 mm caliber (Richard Wolf GmbH, Knittlingen).

2.12.2 Patient Preparation

As for laparoscopy: doxepin HCl, 25 mg IM, on the preceding night and 2 h prior to the examination; 1 h later, meperidine HCl, 75–100 mg IM. Atropine sulfate 0.5 mg SC, at the time of pancreas biopsy and two more doses on the day of examination; the same dose is given three times daily until serum and urine amylase have returned to normal.

2.12.3 Postprocedure Care

Serum amylase and 24-h urinary amylase output daily until within normal range; atropine sulfate, 0.5 mg SC, three times daily until then. The patient need not be fasting.

2.12.4 Technique

2.12.4.1 Inspection

The head of the pancreas can be seen without difficulty with the patient lying on his left side and the head of the table slightly raised, unless the major omentum is thickened by an excessive amount of fat. Ideally, the major omentum is transparent, causing the pancreas to appear as though it were situated intraperitoneally when viewed from a distance. The thin, bright red, and tortuous omental vessels are only visible upon close inspection and can be displaced relative to the fixed pancreas. The yellow-orange pancreatic parenchyma can be differentiated from adipose tissue by the absence of a glistening sheen, typical of the latter [2]. The pancreas follows the outline of the duodenal C loop where, typically, two to three blood vessels, the size of a drinking straw, emerge from the medial wall of the descending duodenum and cross the pancreatic head (Fig. 1). The palpation probe is introduced about two fingerbreadths above and to the right of the umbilicus and is used to determine consistency and mobility of the organ. When the major omentum contains only a moderate amount of fat, it is manipulated with the probe until a transparent area is found through which the head of the pancreas can be inspected piece by piece.

The body of the pancreas is inspected in a similar fashion. This part of the pancreoscopy occurs through the minor omentum, which frequently contains little fat and is transparent near the lesser gastric curvature of older patients. In these cases, large parts of the pancreatic body and tail can be visualized. The patient is in the right lateral decubitus position and the head of the table is elevated. The lateral part of the left hepatic lobe frequently has to be moved out of the way with the "back side" of the side-viewing instrument to gain sufficient distance from the lesser gastric curvature and the pancreas [3]. The palpation probe is best introduced medially and cranially to the laparoscope, about one fingerbreadth left to the midline and one fingerbreadth caudal to the lower costal margin or the xiphoid.

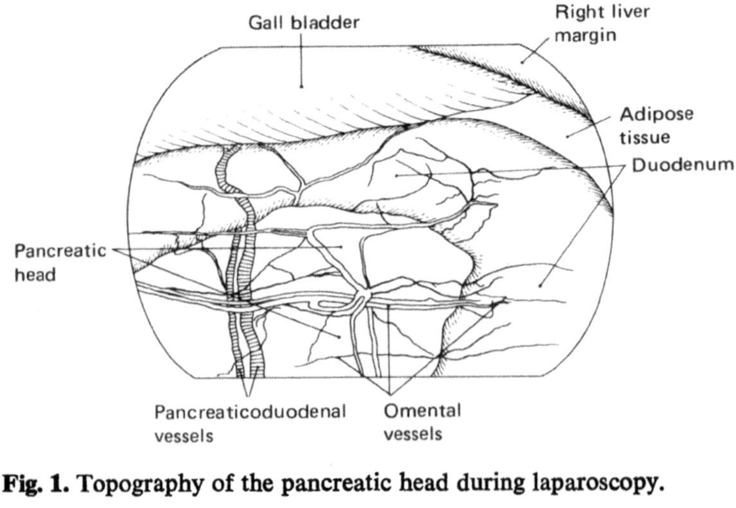

Fig. 1. Topography of the pancreatic head during laparoscopy.

This permits the usual practice of guiding the laparoscope with the right hand and performing manipulations with the left.

Photographic documentation of the pancreatic head and body presents no problems if the patient is positioned as described. The photographs will also show the accessory instruments in use.

Direct pancreoscopy and biopsy after penetration of the major omentum by the laparoscope and "bursoscopy" through the foramen of Winslow represent theoretically attractive possibilities for evaluation of the entire pancreas and the posterior wall of the stomach [4], but this technique did not gain practical significance. Japanese authors recently described a new two-channel laparoscope [1]. The lesser omentum first is penetrated by two forceps introduced through the scope, which is then advanced into the lesser omental sac, allowing inspection of the pancreas and performance of directed target biopsies.

2.12.4.2 Biopsy

Due to the large number and variable course of the pancreatic excretory ducts, the pancreatic head should be biopsied with a forceps consisting of two cupped jaws rather than with the Menghini needle. Only when enlargement and induration of the head of the pancreas strongly suggest the presence of carcinoma may fine needle aspiration be carried out to obtain material for cytologic evaluation (see p. 49). The biopsy forceps yields particles sufficiently large for histologic interpretation at low risk to the patient.

The first step consists of using the scissors to incise both leaves of the major omentum for about 5 mm to keep the forceps from sliding off the peritoneum (Fig. 2).

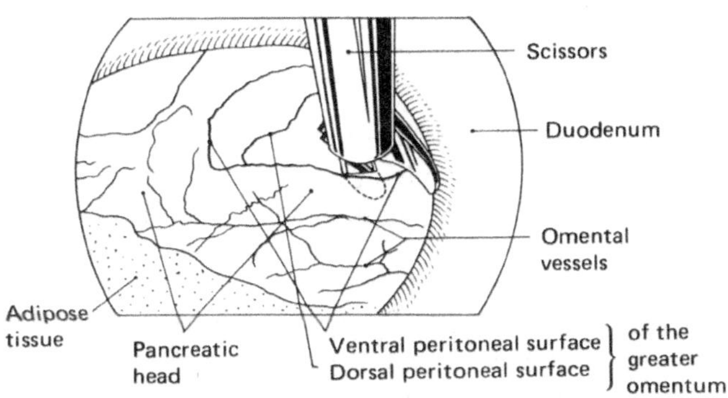

Fig. 2. Incision of both leaves of the greater omentum.

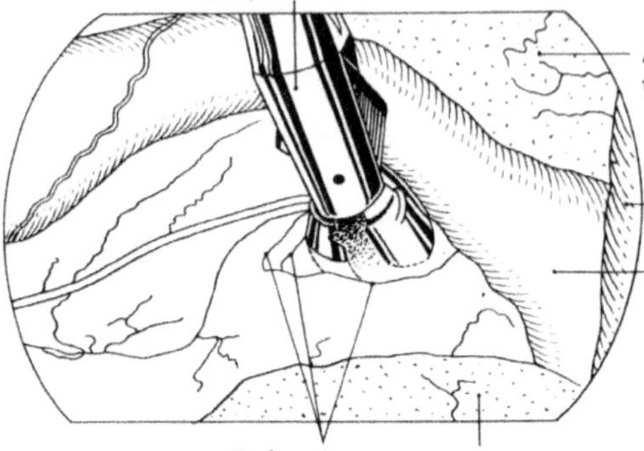

Fig. 3. Biopsy of the exposed pancreas with the two-jaw forceps.

The forceps is half-opened and two or three particles are obtained. Flexible endoscopic biopsy forceps with a central fixation spike may also be employed. Bleeding is minimal in most cases (Fig. 3).

Immediately following the biopsy procedure, we instill aprotinin (Trasylol, 500,000 units) with a 20-cm needle between the pancreatic head and major omentum. Pancreatic biopsy, including incision of the omentum, is usually painless. At most, the patient experiences a brief, sharp pain when the closed forceps is pulled back.

The body of the pancreas may be biopsied as above and fine needle aspirations may also be performed for cytodiagnosis. Thin Menghini needles have also been used successfully. The Menghini needle should, however, only be inserted into markedly thickened and prominent portions of the organ because the normally soft pancreatic tissue is easily penetrated with attendant risk of injury to dorsally situated organs, such as the aorta and left kidney.

2.12.5 Indications

Inspection of the pancreas should be attempted during each laparoscopy. Evaluation of the pancreatic head and body are to be considered part of any comprehensive laparoscopic examination, unless the organ is obscured by fat in the omentum. The examination time is hardly lengthened, even when the palpation probe has to be inserted.

The value of laparoscopic *pancreatic biopsy* is often overestimated, especially in the context of histologic or cytologic confirmation of carcinoma. Laparoscopic biopsy is not very useful for the early diagnosis of operable pancreatic carcinoma. The reason for this is the fact that 60%–70% of pancreatic cancers arise in the center of the pancreatic head and the rest deep in the body and tail. These areas are out of reach of the biopsy forceps. Tumors that have penetrated to the anterior surface of the organ before metastasizing are, unfortunately, rare exceptions. When early carcinoma is suspected or when the pancreas appears abnormal during laparoscopy, duodenoscopy with retrograde pancreatography, combined with cytologic study of aspirated pancreatic secretions (pp. 74 and 52), is the method of choice.

Chronic recurrent pancreatitis of uncertain etiology, causing exocrine pancreatic insufficiency, is diagnosed more reliably by a pancreozymin-secretin test and, possibly, endoscopic retrograde pancreatography than by laparoscopic pancreatic biopsy.

The indications for pancreatic biopsy are limited, in our opinion, to the histologic confirmation of recurrent sclerosing pancreatitis of the alcoholic and of pancreatic siderosis in patients with hemochromatosis. These diagnoses cannot be obtained by any other method.

2.12.6 Contraindications

Biopsy is contraindicated when clinical observations and laboratory results suggest acute pancreatitis and when the pancreas is found to be greatly enlarged and congested. Bleeding disorders dictate the same caution as with liver biopsy. Pancreatic biopsy is unnecessary in the presence of liver metastases and occlusion of bile ducts by tumor.

2.12.7 Complications

No complications have occurred, provided the prophylactic measures outlined above were observed. Serum and urinary amylase, however, rise to abnormal values in about 50% of patients after pancreatic biopsy. These changes regularly revert to normal within a few days. Pain radiating from the epigastrium to both flanks rarely occurs after biopsy and responds to analgesic medication.

References

1. Ishida, H., Kanazawa, H., Furukawa, Y., Kuroda, H., Kobayashi, M., Tsuneoka, K.: The inspection and aimed biopsy of the pancreas by the new type of laparoscope. IV. World Congress of Digestive Endoscopy, Madrid 1978
2. Look, D., Henning, H., Lüders, C. J.: Darstellung und Biopsie des Pankreaskopfes bei der Laparoskopie. Z. Gastroenterol. *10*, 109 (1972)
3. Meyer-Burg, J.: The inspection, palpation and biopsy of the pancreas by peritoneoscopy. Endoscopy *4*, 99 (1972)
4. Strauch, M., Lux, G., Ottenjann, R.: Infragastric pancreoscopy. Endoscopy *5*, 30 (1973)

2.13

Fiberendoscopy of the Common Bile and the Major Pancreatic Duct

M. CLASSEN

2.13.1 Fibercholedochoscopy

About 8%–30% of stones remain in the common bile duct after operations for choledocholithiasis [4]. This rate can be reduced to 0–3% by use of operative cholangioscopy [4]. A newly developed method permits inspection of the bile duct system by the peroral route [2,3].

2.13.1.1 Instruments

Flexible choledochoscopes (e.g., model CHF, Olympus) are now available in addition to the existing rigid cholangioscopes that were introduced by Wildegans in 1953. The image is transmitted through a fiberglass bundle and the cold light through two light transmission bundles. The instrumentation channel is used for irrigation and retrieval of biopsies. The optical field is 60°, the focal depth 3–50 mm.

For peroral cholangioscopy, a thin (2-mm) fiberendoscope is introduced through the instrumentation channel of the duodenoscope and manipulated through the papilla of Vater into the common bile duct.

2.13.1.2 Technique

Intraoperative cholangioscopy is carried out through an incision of the choledochus during laparotomy. The instrument is introduced through an irrigation cannula, and the common bile duct is occluded by an inflatable cuff. Irrigation fluid can be aspirated from this closed system without risk of flooding the operative field [5].

The optical qualities of the CHF cholangioscope are good; its flexibility allows inspection of the entire bile duct system up to the second-order ducts. In the opposite direction, the duodenum can be entered through the papilla of Vater; occasionally, the carefully advanced biopsy forceps has to serve as a guide. Stone retrieval forceps are not yet available; the theoretical possibility exists, however, to use a Fogarty catheter for this purpose.

The cholangioscope (baby scope), which is introduced into the choledochus through the duodenoscope (mother scope), permits retrograde inspection up to the second-order bile ducts during peroral cholangioscopy. The available prototypes, however, have not yet achieved the quality needed for routine use.

2.13.1.3 Complications

Complications of fiberoptic cholangioscopy, such as bile duct perforation, rupture of the common bile duct suture line, or cholangitis, have not yet been observed.

2.13.2 Endoscopy of the Pancreatic Duct (Pancreaticoscopy; Wirsungoscopy)

During laparotomy, the pancreatic duct can be inspected in a descending direction after removal of the tail of the organ, or in ascending direction through the papilla of Vater [1]. Preliminary results of peroral pancreaticoscopy have been published [2].

2.13.2.1 Instrumentation and Technique

For intraoperative pancreaticoscopy, a very thin endoscope (e.g., bronchoscope BF-3A; Olympus) of 3.2-mm diameter is employed when the duct of Wirsung is of normal caliber. The tip of the instrument can be deflected upward by 180° and downward by 30°. The choledochofiberscope CHF, type B, described above, can be used when the pancreatic duct system is dilated. The thin bronchoscope does not contain an extra channel; irrigation during the examination has to occur through a 1-mm plastic catheter that is introduced into the duct with the endoscope. Sterile physiologic saline solution is perfused continuously and is aspirated as it exits from the duct. The same prototype as for peroral cholangioscopy is used for peroral pancreaticoscopy.

2.13.2.2 Indications

The differentiation between chronic pancreatitis and carcinoma of the pancreas is the most important indication. Even ERCP yields only indirect radiologic findings that do not allow definitive conclusions to be drawn. Endoscopy with the capabilities of obtaining biopsies under direct vision represents a promising approach in view of the fact that 90% of pancreatic carcinomis originate from ductal epithelium.

Attempts are in progress to improve the prototypes of the "mother-baby" endoscope. This combination should eventually permit the routine transpapillary inspection of bile and pancreatic ducts.

References

1. Classen, M., Schwemmle, K., Demling, L.: Endoscopy of the pancreatic duct. Endoscopy *4*, 221–223 (1972)
2. Kawai, K., Nakajina, M., Akasaka, J., Shimamotu, K., Murakami, K.: Eine neue endoskopische Technik: Die perorale Choledocho-Pancreatic-oskopie. Leber Magen Darm *6*, 121–124 (1976)
3. Rösch, W., Koch, H., Demling, L.: Peroral cholangioscopy. Endoscopy *8*, 172–175 (1976)
4. Schaudig, A., Lukas, M., v. Bary, S.: Erste Erfahrungen mit einem verbesserten Cholangioskop. In: Fortschritte der Endoskopie. Ottenjann, R. (Ed.), Vol. IV. Stuttgart: Schattauer 1973
5. Wiendl, H. J., Piger, A.: Erste Erfahrungen mit einem neuen flexiblen Choledochoskop bein Eingriffen an den Gallenwegen. In: Fortschritte der Endoskopie. Ottenjann, R. (Ed.), Vol. IV. Stuttgart: Schattauer 1973

2.14

Laparoscopic Splenoportography

L. WANNAGAT

In 1951, two young Italian surgeons, Abeatici and Campi, of Doggliotti's school, developed a method in experimental animals in which contrast material is injected percutaneously into the spleen under radiologic observation with consequent visualization of the portal circulation [1]. One year later, the French surgeon, Leger, applied this method to patients. Radiologists prefer this "blind" splenoportography to this day although, regardless of other technical refinements, the splenic puncture occurs without direct visual control.

Laparoscopic splenoportography has some decided advantages [1]. The patient is able to breathe freely during the entire procedure. There are no time constraints. The patient lies in a movable cradle, horizontal, and on his right side. Depending on the situation, the head of the table may have to be raised or lowered. Used in this fashion, the method yields reliable information on liver structure and the hemodynamic status of the portal circulation. Prolonged registration of intrasplenic pressure provides important clues to the load capacity and functional characteristics of the portal circulatory system. The selection of photographic documentation should be flexible and adapted to the situation encountered. The diagnosis of hepatofugal or zero net flow in the portal vein is of great importance for diagnosis, prophylaxis, and therapy of intrahepatic causes of portal hypertension, as well as of portal and splenic vein thrombosis. This information can be obtained by exposing serial X-ray films for up to 10 min after injection. Spleen size is determined visually in different positions, and splenic function is evaluated by pharmocokinetic means. The spleen may be punctured nine times or more during one session when each of the three splenic segments needs to be studied repeatedly. Further specialized procedures may be added, such as segmental porto-, veno-, and arteriography and selective lymphangiography [2]. Photographic contrast and quality are excellent in the presence of a pneumoperitoneum. Electrocoagulation needs to be available in the event of severe bleeding.

2.14.1 Instruments

Instruments and method as described in Sect. 2.11. Before creating the pneumoperitoneum, we use a needle (length 15 cm, diameter 0.8 mm) to gain spatial orientation in the abdomen by palpation. This has proven valuable in the presence of highly vascular adhesions and of portal collateral circulation and helps avoid penetrating injuries and bleeding. Our experience is based on 10,042 laparoscopies. Next, the actual pneu needle (length 10 cm, diameter 1 mm; with stylet and double channel in the shaft) is introduced. Other equipment consists of splenic puncture needle (length 17 cm; diameter 1.2 mm; distal 5 cm graduated at intervals of 1 or 2 cm); special applicator sticks (Wolf, Knittlingen); electrocoagulation probe: Siemens Sireskop radiologic unit with removable rotating cradle and rapid film changer.

2.14.2 Patient Preparation

Clear liquids and enema on the evening before. Immediately prior to examination: 20 mg Pantopon IM, 10 mg diazepam IV, and 50 mg promethazine HCl IM.

2.14.3 Postprocedure Care

For the following night: a suppository containing 60 mg aprobarbital and 600 mg phenacetin; 600 mg phenacetin and scopolamine HBr, as needed; white blood cell count, recording of pulse and temperature at frequent intervals. Diet: clear liquids on the day of examination; the following day, gruel for breakfast, soup for lunch, soft diet for supper and on the next day. Regular diet thereafter.

2.14.4 Technique

The patient is supine; he may be turned on his left or right side in the movable cradle. The head of the table may have to be raised up to 45°, especially when the spleen is difficult to visualize due to fixation by adhesions or to lateral extension of an unusually large left hepatic lobe. The puncture is made at the medial margin of the organ, aiming at the center of the middle or caudal segment, to a depth of 4–5 cm (Fig. 1a, b). The cannula should not be introduced near the hilum because of the concentration of large arteries and veins in that area. The anterior (ventral) approach has the disadvantage that the needle may penetrate the posterior capsule with consequent injection of contrast medium into the retro- or parasplenic space and eventual appearance in the peritoneal cavity. Use of the cranial segment should be the exception rather than the rule. The proximity of the dome of the diaghragm brings with it the danger of pneumothorax or of a circumscribed reactive pleuritis.

The *decholin* (dehydrocholate Na) *test* yields initial information on the portal circulation [3]. A positive test indicates that the needle is situated properly within the spleen. The arm-tongue time is determined on the day prior to the laparoscopy: the interval between injection of 5 ml decholin Na (20%) into an antecubital vein and appearance of a bitter taste. The spleen-tongue time is obtained during splenic puncture. The "portal time" is the difference between the spleen-tongue and arm-tongue times. The bitter taste normally is experienced within 25–40 s following injection. It may take as long as 60 s. A negative test is defined as the absence of any bitter sensation within 60 s. The lips and tongue should be kept moist. The spleen-tongue time is abnormally brief in the presence of collateral circulation, of a spontaneous splenorenal shunt, and with hepatofugal portal flow. In these situations, the portal time may be zero or, occasionally, achieve a negative value. A negative spleen-tongue time (no bitter taste within 60 s) may be an expression of the functional autonomy of different spleen segments or, if reproducible, it may reflect true portal stasis with secondary splenic insufficiency, such as fibroadenomatosis or splenic decompensation according to Ewerbeck [3]. The spleen-tongue time may also be negative due to the dynamic regulation of the splenic circulation, in the absence of organic changes. In this situation, the test typically becomes positive when repeated within 20 min or less. When the venous part of the terminal splenic circulation is closed with the arterial sphincters either open or closed, [filling and storage phase of Knisely, 1936, 3], the test will be negative. The test records positively as soon as, either, the streaming phase (in- and outflow open) or the emptying phase (inflow closed, outflow open) begin [3].

A second precautionary measure to assure successful splenoportography is the preliminary injection of 5 ml of Conray contrast medium. The main injection follows immediately if no side-effects are reported and the television monitor shows steady disappearance of the contrast material from the spleen. The main injection may be repeated three or four times, utilizing the other splenic segments as well, as indicated (Fig. 2). Withdrawal of the needle should occur slowly and should be completed only when blood no longer trickles along the outside of the cannula. Electro-

a

b

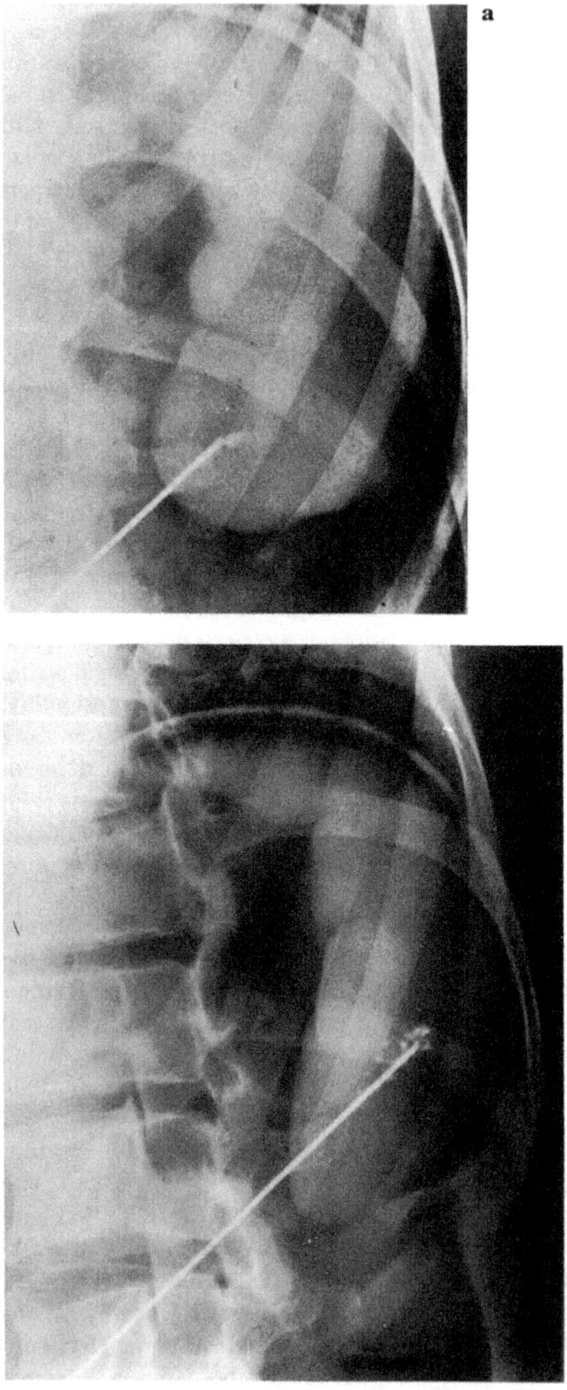

Fig. 1, a–b. Laparoscopic splenoportography; **a** incorrectly positioned cannula; **b** correctly positioned cannula.

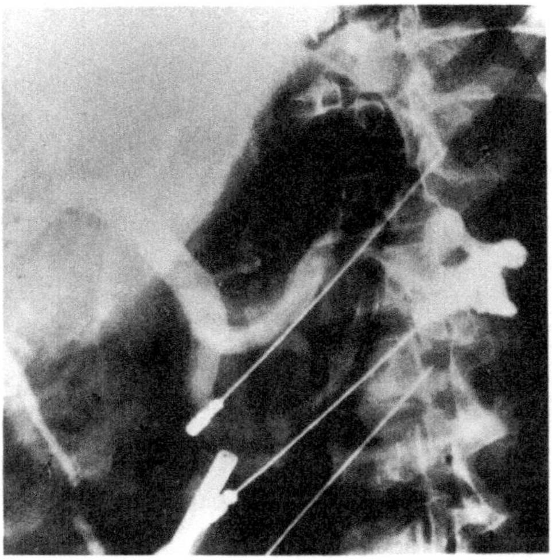

Fig. 2. Simultaneous multiple puncture; three cannulas in the spleen (cranial, middle and caudal segment).

coagulation is used only in case the bleeding is massive and unremitting. It is important to realize that pseudoarterial bleeding may be observed for up to 10 min during the filling phase (open inflow, closed outflow) and the streaming phase (in- and outflow open). This type of bleeding is not nearly as dramatic as true arterial bleeding (pulsating blood jets up to 3 cm high) and, in contrast to the latter, subsides spontaneously at the moment of phase change (from filling or streaming phase to storage or emptying phase).

2.14.5 Indications

1) Diagnosis and prognosis of portal hypertension
2) Indication for porto-systemic shunt
3) Determination of the functional and hemodynamic characteristics of the portal circulation
4) Differential diagnosis of masses in the upper abdomen

The most important parameter for documentation of *portal hypertension* is the transhepatic registration of portal venous pressure during *segmental portography* [2]. A graduated cannula is introduced to a depth of 4–6 cm into the central portion of that hepatic segment that exhibits the greatest vascularization during splenoportography. Normal values are between 10 and 15 mm Hg; values exceeding 20 mm Hg signify portal hypertension. A precise reference point is a prerequisite for exact pressure determination. This is achieved in the same fashion as for splenic pulp pressure measurement (Fig. 3): The parallelogram principle is applied

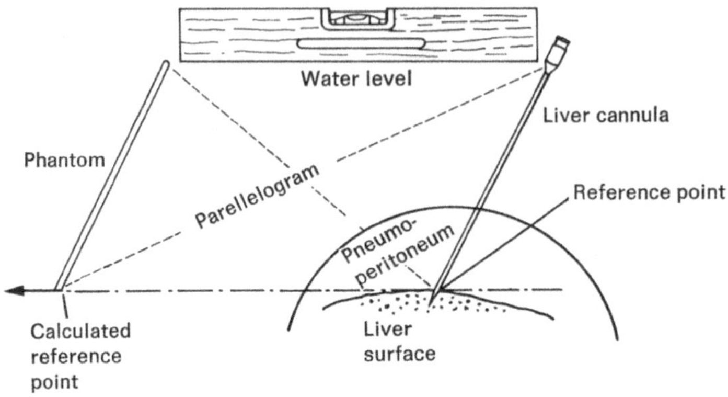

Fig. 3. Parallelogram principle to measure portal venous pressure.

with use of a Statham element and an electronic-photographic recording device. Measurements taken at different points differ by less than 1 mm Hg; possible sources of error are discussed in [4]. The demonstration of partial or complete hepatofugal blood flow in the portal system is nearly as important as the direct diagnosis of portal hypertension. Filling of the coronary veins by contrast material confirms the presence of esophageal varices. The radiologic finding of an immobile contrast column near the spleen (duration of up to 9 min after start of injection) is very significant and can easily be differentiated from stasis of contrast material due to functional causes. In the latter case, the contrast will slowly start flowing toward the liver after 10–30 s, coincident with a phase change in the splenic circulation.

Hepatofugal flow and an immobile contrast column as a consequence of an intrahepatic block are certain signs of portal hypertension. The degree of hypertension, however, is best assessed by measurement during segmental portography. An enlarged, spongy spleen and splenic fibrosis are important clues for the presence of portal hypertension, provided splenic vein occlusion (thrombosis) can be excluded.

Absolute indications for porto-systemic shunt operation are (1) the combination of portal pressure (recorded transhepatically) of 28 mm Hg with hepatofugal blood flow, and (2) preceding bleeding from esophageal varices together with either one of these parameters. A *prophylactic shunt* should be considered in the following situations: (1) equal values of splenic pulp pressure during the streaming phase and transhepatic portal pressure (stasis); (2) immobile contrast column, spontaneous splenorenal shunt (16 among 3620 splenoportographies), decompensated Cruveilhier-Baumgarten syndrome, or prominent arteriovenous anastomoses near the splenic hilum in the presence of documented portal hypertension; (3) occasionally, a leathery, cirrhotic liver with lymphectasia (documented by selective lymphangiography) and ascites; (4) distal splenic vein thrombosis with occlusion of the coronary veins leading to engorgement of esophageal veins; (5) occlusion or atresia of the portal vein as indication for splenorenal anastomosis.

The *functional properties of the portal system* can only be evaluated by dynamic and varied use of splenoportography [1]. Changes in position revealing orthostatic effects, the streaming phenomenon (indentation of the contrast column at the inflow point of contributory veins), and layering of the contrast material in vessels taking a horizontal course, all indicate slowing of the portal circulation.

Liver tumors cannot be detected by this technique until they have reached a size of 2–3 cm. Splenoportography contributes mainly to the diagnosis of extrahepatic masses in the upper abdomen. The Budd-Chiari syndrome can be recognized only at an advanced state when the thrombotic process has extended to the portal system. Early stages of this syndrome can reliably be detected by segmental porto- or venography (Fig. 4). Abrupt termination of blood vessels, not to be confused with vasospasm, is the result of inflammatory processes and is an important residual of viral hepatitis. Hepatic proliferation of fibroconnective tissue is impressively reflected by fibrotic stenosis of large portal vein branches; the "tree root" phenomenon [1], with better visualization of branch veins than of the larger afferent veins, is another manifestation of this process. Splenoportography is of little value in assessing the course of hepatitis, i.e., in differentiating between self-limited and chronic forms and developing cirrhosis.

2.14.6 Contraindications

The same reservations apply as to laparoscopy in general, although we pay little attention to the prothrombin time. Experience has shown that the prothrombin time of splenic and hepatic blood may be much less prolonged than in peripheral blood. In addition, most bleeding episodes from liver and spleen can be terminated by electrocoagulation. Technical problems arise when an enlarged left hepatic lobe prevents splenic puncture and when dense adhesions have pulled the spleen up toward the diaphragm or even prevent visualization of the organ altogether. We follow the motto, "Always risk an attempt." The abdomen bearing the scars of multiple operations often provides no obstacle to splenoportography, while the procedure may be found impossible in a "virgin" abdomen. The soft, septic spleen, splenic infarcts and metastases, and involvement by leukemia are relative contraindications. Obviously, the method cannot be employed in the asplenic patient and in those cases where the spleen is invisible or unreachable even with the patient on his right side and in near vertical position (phrenico-

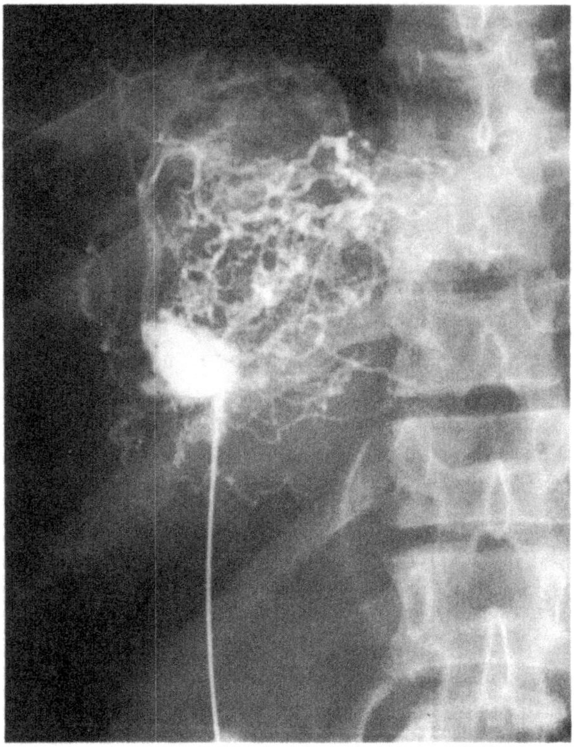

Fig. 4. M.W., 34 years. Segmental portography, Budd-Chiari syndrome. Convoluted portal venous pathways; no hepatic veins; one normal portal vein branch close to the lateral segment boundary.

colic ligament widened by adhesions; markedly distended small or large intestine; excessively respiratory excursion of the spleen). Our rate of failed attempts is 3% among 3620 cases; with the percutaneous blind technique (not hindered by adhesions) it is 2% [Roesch in 1].

2.14.7 Complications

Splenic rupture (0 = No. in our patient material), subcapsular hematoma (52), and large intrasplenic hematomas (521) are the direct result of the technique which features contrast material injection into the splenic parenchyma rather than intravascularly. Puncture of the splenic artery (0), perforation of the spleen (2), and injury to adjacent organs (0) are rare when the laparoscopic approach is chosen. On one occasion, the caudal pole of the spleen was injured by the trocar; the alarming bleeding could be stopped by electrocoagulation. Pseudocomplications: brief, pulsating bleeding after withdrawal of the cannula, resulting from the phasic changes in splenic circulation (see above), cannot be attributed to faulty technique. Blood loss may be considerable and transfusion (one case) may be necessary. These pseudoarterial bleeding episodes occur mainly with advanced cirrhosis in which the arterial sphincters of the terminal circulation often become insufficient, the so-called arterialization phenomenon [3]. The spleen responds to portal hypertension by increasing the pulp pressure to maintain blood flow in the face of significant intrahepatic blockade.

Conclusion. The risk of laparoscopic splenoportography is considerably smaller than that of the classic percutaneous approach. Additional advantages include better quality of the radiographs, the possibility of individualizing the procedure, the lack of time pressure, and the ability to extend the examination by the use of additional procedures. Hence, laparoscopic splenoportography is the method of choice for evaluation and diagnosis of the extrahepatic portal circulation. Intrahepatic alterations are better demonstrated by segmental veno-, port-, and arteriography, by selective lymphangiography, and by developing biochemical methods, including the use of radioactive isotopes.

References

1. WANNAGAT, L.: Splenoportografie. Leber Magen Darm *3*, 3 (1973)
2. WANNAGAT, L.: Die Segmentangiographie der Leber mit laparoskopischer Technik und Elektrokoagulation
3. WANNAGAT, L.: Autonomy of splenic segments. Stuttgart: Thieme (in press)
4. WANNAGAT, L.: Druckmessung und Röntgendarstellung der Pfortader. In: Klinische Hepatologie. KÜHN, H. H., v. OLDERSHAUSEN, H. F., WERNZE, H. (Ed.). Stuttgart: Thieme (in press)

2.15
Laparoscopic Cholecystography

L. WANNAGAT

Direct *cholecysto-cholangiography* by the laparoscopic approach was developed simultaneously by Royer, a South American, and Lee, a North American. The publications appeared 1 year later in 1942 [3]. Credit for originating this method should, therefore, go to both investigators. Henning, Demling, and associates began to use this technique in Germany in 1952. The main advantage of this method is that pure, undiluted bile can be obtained for microscopic, bacteriologic, and chemical analyses. Structure and function of the gallbladder are determined radiologically while only limited information about the bile ducts is obtained. *Transhepatic cholangio-cholecystography* can be performed at the same time and gives detailed views of the biliary duct system [2]. Our experience is based on 2395 direct punctures of the gallbladder and on 147 laparoscopic transhepatic cholangiographies.

2.15.1 Instruments

Same as for laparoscopy (see p. 142). Additional equipment: one pointed needle, 15 cm long and 0.8 mm external diameter, graduated at 1–2 cm intervals; one special swab (Wolf, Knittlingen), 33 cm long, 3 mm diameter; one suction tube with lateral openings and closed at the distal end, 29 cm long, 3 mm diameter (Wolf, Knittlingen); and one aspiration pump (Vacutron 4012, Kleinknecht, Erlangen) with tubing and collection bottle (Figs. 1 and 2).

2.15.2 Patient Preparation

Same as for splenoportography (p. 166).

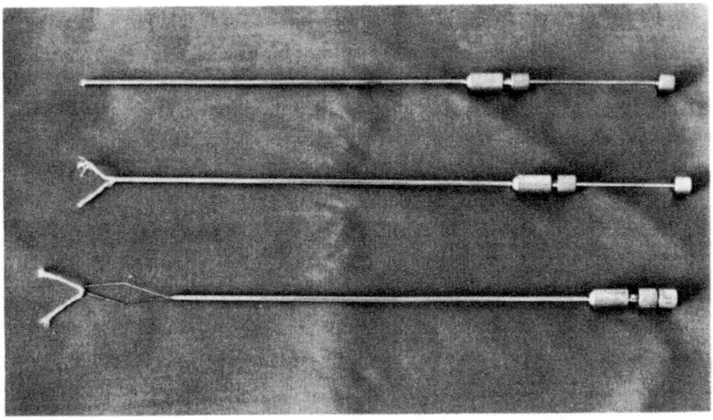

Fig. 1. Swab: *above*, ready for use; *below*, open with cotton wool threaded into place.

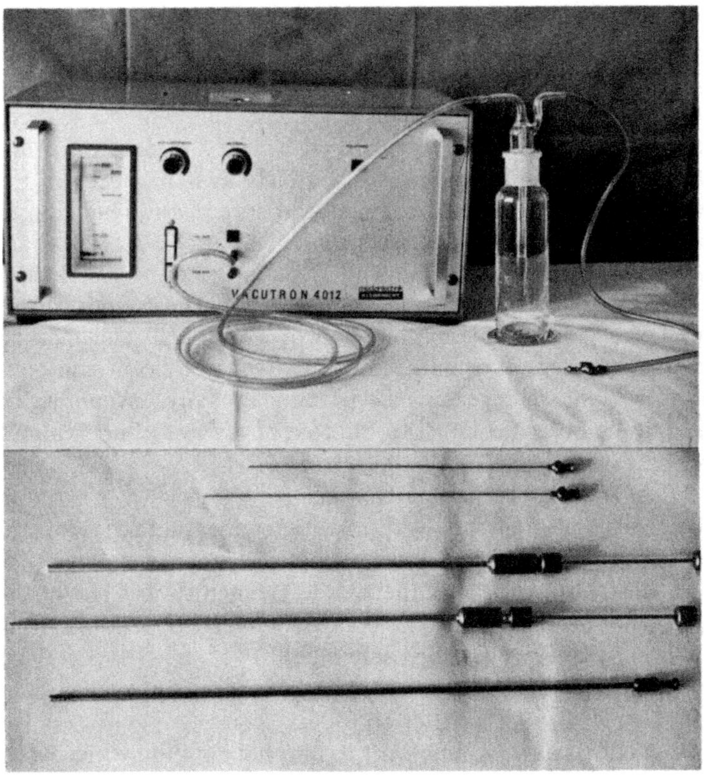

Fig. 2. Suction pump with collecting bottle, cannulas, swab, and suction tube.

2.15.3 Postprocedure Care

The patient should remain supine for 24 h. Mild analgesics for abdominal pain without findings of peritoneal irritation; oral hygiene; sips of warm tea; intravenous fluids as needed. Antibiotics when cholangitis or bacteremia are suspected, e.g., doxycycline hyclate IV. The clips are removed after 2 days when the patient may return to full activity.

2.15.4 Technique

The laparoscope is inserted first at the usual place, left and caudal to the umbilicus. Next, a smaller trocar is introduced at the lower liver margin, roughly between the gallblader and ligamentum teres. It is used for liver biopsy and for the accessory instruments (palpation and electrocoagulation probes, forceps, applicator stick). The gallbladder can now be punctured, provided it is in full view. If not, attempts have to be made to remove or circumvent the intervening structures: Omentum or intestine are moved aside or the liver is elevated with the palpation probe or the applicator stick until the organ is fully visible at the concave liver surface. In the presence of adhesions, one tries to dissect a small window, exposing part of the gallbladder surface. Following local anesthesia, the cannula is advanced at an angle of about 45° to the abdominal wall with the needle tip impinging without tension or angulation on a relatively avascular area of the gallbladder serosa. The preferred site is the medial aspect at the junction of the corpus and neck because the needle tract closes best in this location. The organ becomes difficult to see following aspiration of the gallbladder bile (tobacco pouch shape) through the lateral wall. The fundus is not suitable for puncture because the combination of a thin wall and marked distention increases the risk that the needle tract will not close with consequent uncontrolled bile spillage into the peritoneal cavity. A number of precautions have to be observed to assure success of the procedure without complications:

a) The puncture should be made with a short, sudden, and vigorous motion, taking care to avoid penetration of the posterior wall. Slow and steady advancing of the needle frequently just indents the organ without penetrating the wall or moves the gallbladder aside, especially when it is not tensely filled.
b) The gallbladder should be nearly empty before the needle is withdrawn.
c) In older patients it is very important to aim for an oblique needle tract through the wall. After the needle has been withdrawn, the site should be carefully massaged with the applicator stick to help

occlude the tract in order to decrease the risk of a bile leak. These precautions need not be observed as stringently in young patients in whom the more elastic gallbladder wall tends to close the needle tract efficiently.

d) Thin bile is easily obtained. Thick, viscous bile or bile containing "gravel" frequently has to be aspirated by hand. This may require much time and effort but complete aspiration is essential for avoiding bile leaks. Should the needle slip out accidentally, it has to be reinserted, but the same penetration site should not be used twice.

2.15.5 Indications

Diseases of the gallbladder that cannot be fully delineated by routine clinical methods: calculi, adenomata, papillomas, hydrops, porcelain- and raspberry gallbladder, milky bile, biliary dyskinesias. Empyemas should be punctured with great care; intravesical and intraperitoneal instillation of antibiotics is required after the pus has been aspirated. The indications may be broadened with increasing experience, especially when a surgical team is available at all times.

The above indications apply also in the presence of septate gallbladder (Phrygian cap), diverticula, Luschka's ducts, external trauma, and pendulous or siphon gallbladder.

Laparoscopic cholecystography can also add to the differential diagnosis and prognostic evaluation of patients with chronic hepatitis and cirrhosis by providing bile for chemical analysis [2]. Patients with identical appearance of cirrhosis on liver biopsy may have very different rehabilitation potential and prognosis, depending on the appearance of their bile. Dark-brown to brown-black concentrated bile in a blue-green colored, moderately distended gallbladder is a favorable finding. Thin, dyscholic bile, usually found in a tightly distended organ, is abnormal.

A flaccid, partly filled gallbladder of grey-white appearance and with thickening of the serosa is typical for advanced intrahepatic cholestasis. Extrahepatic biliary obstruction is signified by the Courvoisier-Terrier syndrome

2.15.6 Contraindications

All contraindications to laparoscopy in general apply. In addition: absence of the gallbladder; gallbladders that cannot be visualized nor reached; gallbladders that cannot be punctured because they are small, collapsed, or unusually mobile; or a shrunken organ containing stones that adhere closely to the wall. The restless and the overly pain-sensitive patient may also cause the examination to fail.

2.15.7 Complications

Bile leaking from the needle tract into the peritoneum is by far the most common complication. Sterile bile causes a chemical peritonitis, infected bile a diffuse bacterial peritonitis. Bile leaks develop:

a) When the needle penetrates the anterior and posterior wall of the gallbladder and the posterior penetration remains open after repositioning of the needle but before the bile is aspirated
b) When the needle slips out of the organ before the gallbladder has been emptied or when the needle tract is placed in a poorly contractile portion of the wall
c) Occasionally, when the gallbladder is overdistended and bile exits along the needle shaft

In all these situations the gallbladder contents must be completely aspirated as promptly as possible and spilled bile should be removed by suction.

While injury to adjacent organs is theoretically possible, the incidence approaches zero, provided the described technique is meticulously adhered to and the examiner is an experienced gastroenterologist-endoscopist.

The formation of wall hematomas causes bleeding to stop in nearly all instances; severe bleeding usually can be terminated by massaging the gallbladder wall with the applicator stick or palpation probe.

Among 2780 procedures reported in the literature until 1976, the complication rate was 0.4%. In our own experience of 2395 laparoscopic cholecystographies we observed two major complications: one subphrenic abscess occurred at a time when we still used the transhepatic approach as recommended by Kalk and bile peritonitis developed in an elderly patient after puncture of the fundus of the gallbladder when the somewhat overdistended organ refilled with bile. Both patients recovered after surgical intervention. Wildhirt reported four instances of bile peritonitis among 150 cases, with two fatal outcomes. This author had also employed the transhepatic approach.

Transhepatic cholangio-cholecystography by the *laparoscopic* approach, with *electrocoagulation* of the puncture site [2], will be mentioned briefly. This method has the advantage over the percutaneous approach described by Carter and Saypol in 1952 in that it can be performed without time constraint. Prior to Carter and Saypol's report, the blind percutaneous approach had been used successfully in three patients in Indochina by

Huard and Do-Xuan-Hop as early as 1931; Lipiodol was used at that time. Timing and detailed strategy of the diagnostic approach can be planned in advance by the examining internist. The laparoscopic approach for study of the intra- and extrahepatic biliary tree has two unique advantages over all other methods, including the "skinny needle" percutaneous method recently reported from Japan: (1) both hepatic lobes (not only the right lobe) can be punctured and (2) the availability of electrocoagulation increases the safety of the procedure.

References

1. WANNAGAT, L.: Die direkte Gallenblasenpunktion mit laparoskopischer Technik. Z. Arztl. Fortbild. (Jena) *52*, issue 11 (1963)
2. WANNAGAT, L.: Die Segmentportographie und die transhepatische Cholangiographie mit laparoskopischer Technik. Vehr. Dtsch. Ges. Inn. Med. *72*, 678 (1967)
3. WANNAGAT, L.: Laparoskopische Cholezystographie und transhepatische Cholangiographie. In: Klinische Gastroenterologie. DEMLING, L. (Ed.), p. 887. Stuttgart: Thieme 1973

2.16

Percutaneous Transhepatic Cholangiography

W. WENZ

Percutaneous transhepatic cholangiography (PTC) is a radiologic method for demonstrating the biliary tract by percutaneous injection of contrast material.

2.16.1 Instruments

A modern radiologic unit with image intensifier, television screen, and motorized tilt table is required. A 10-ml syringe containing procaine HCl 0.5% with a thin needle is needed for local anesthesia. The skin is incised by a disposable scalpel with a blade only a few millimeters long.

The steel puncture needle with Luer-Lok connector is contained in a plastic sheath and is 12 cm long (Longdwel Catheter, Becton, Dickinson & Co., Rutherford, NJ). The metal cannula is withdrawn after the liver has been entered, leaving the flexible plastic catheter in place. Uretero- or colostomy bags may be attached when the catheter is to be used for prolonged biliary decompression.

2.16.2 Patient Preparation

The examination is performed in the morning with the patient kept fasting overnight. He should be told that the liver will be punctured from the side and that he will experience only a pressure sensation in the liver area once the local anesthesia takes effect. Premedication consists of triflupromazine or a combination of meperidine and atropine. The puncture site in the axillary line, 10th intercostal space, is carefully cleaned with iodine solution and draped with sterile towels. Topographic abnormalities of the liver and interposition of gas-filled bowel loops must be excluded by fluoroscopy (Fig. 1).

2.16.3 Postprocedure Care

At the end of the procedure, the contrast medium is reaspirated as far as possible. There is no need to be concerned about the possibility of a bile leak with consequent bile peritonitis, as long as bile flow is found to be unobstructed, i.e., in the absence of mechanical obstructive jaundice. However, when the biliary tract is obstructed, we recommend leaving the plastic catheter in place until surgical decompression is achieved. Surgical intervention immediately following detection of mechanical obstruction is the treatment of choice in any event.

2.16.4 Technique

The caudal liver margin is marked and the area viewed fluoroscopically on the television screen. Local anesthesia with 5–6 ml procaine HCl 0.5% is carried to the parietal peritoneum, aiming at the 12th thoracic vertebra. The skin is incised at the 10th intercostal space in the midaxillary line and the cholangiography needle pointed toward the 12th thoracic vertebra. It is advanced at a slight angle, from lateral-caudal to medial-ventral, to the level of the hilus of the liver. The needle should run in a cranial direction, one to two fingerbreadths above the caudal liver margin. The metal cannula is then removed and the emergence of bile is noted as the plastic catheter is withdrawn slightly. The success rate lies between 80% and 90% (Table 1).

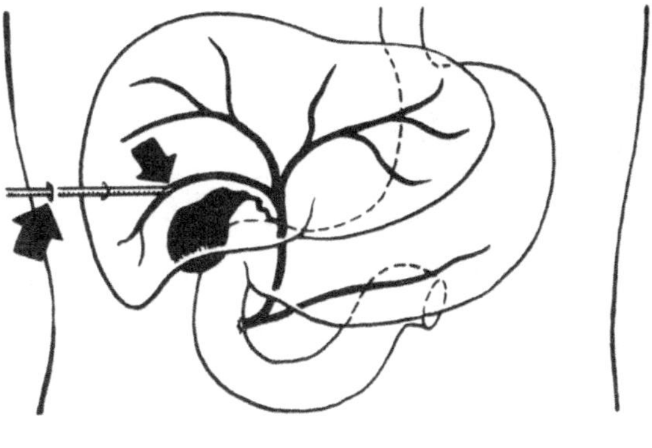

Fig. 1. Technique of transhepatic cholangiography (PTC).

Table 1. Results of 218 successful procedures.

Tumor	129
Stone obstruction	50
Papillary stenosis	9
Stone impacted in the papilla	8
Hepatitis	6
Postoperative stricture	6
Duodenal diverticulum	1
Hepatic cyst	1
Echinococcal cyst	1
Liver metastases	7
Total	218 (success rate about 80%)

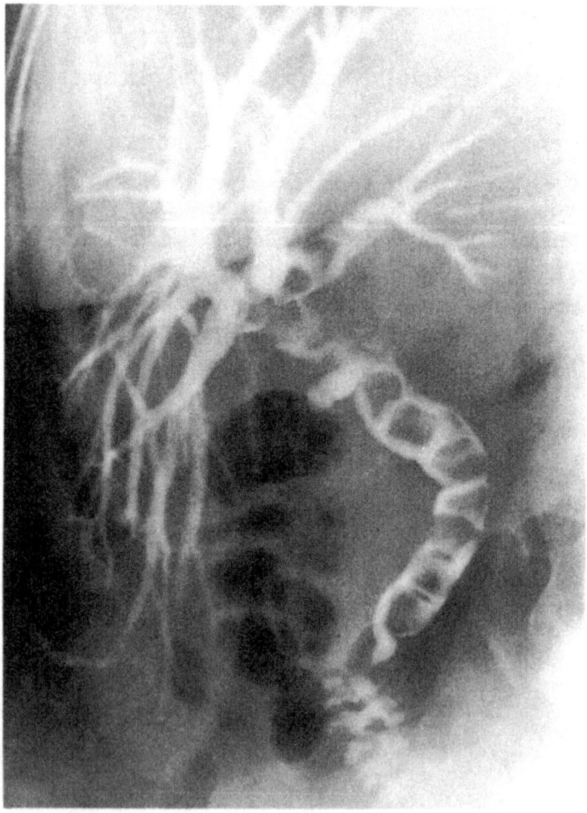

Fig. 2. **PTC**: choledocholithiasis.

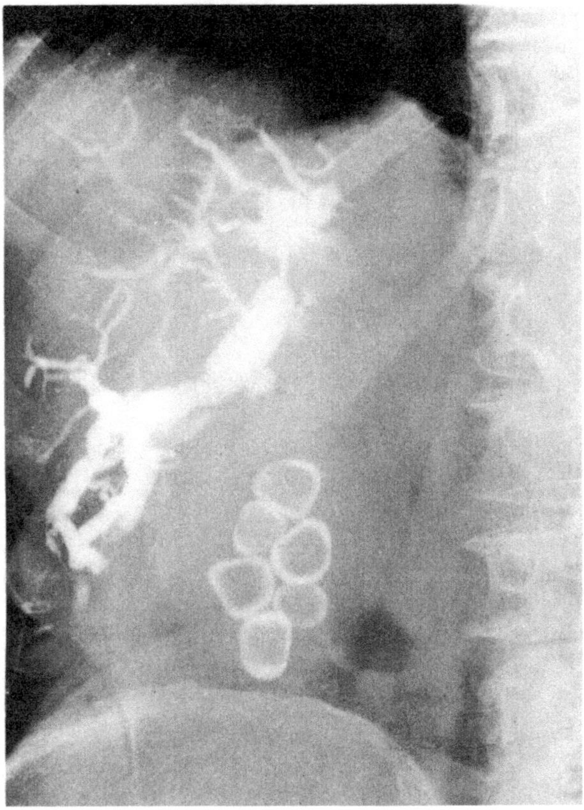

Fig. 3. PTC: intrahepatic bile duct occlusion by carcinoma in presence of pre-existing cholecystolithiasis.

When blood appears from the catheter, a few milliliters of contrast material are injected. With position in a hepatic vein, the material will flow in a cranial-medial direction. A wedge-shaped segment of liver is opacified when a portal vein branch is entered. Puncture of arterial vessels is extremely rare.

The catheter tip continues to be withdrawn slowly until bile begins to drip. As much bile as possible is allowed to drain. Then, 10–30 ml of a dense contrast medium (Urografin 76%) are injected slowly under constant fluoroscopic control, the total volume depending on the capacity of the biliary tree. With the table tilted slightly head-up, the larger bile ducts, including the common bile duct, begin to fill after some time, provided there is no mechanical obstruction.

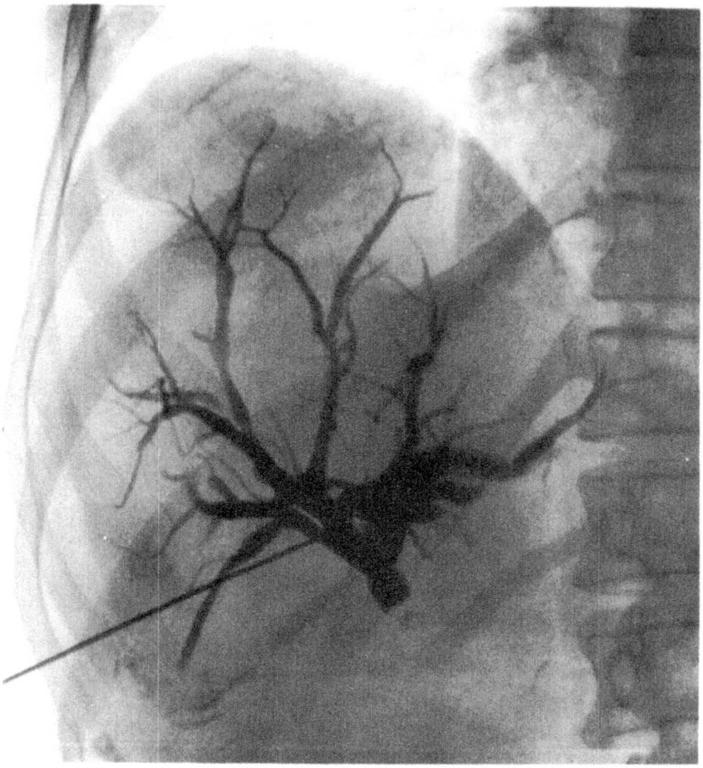

Fig. 4. Common hepatic duct occlusion following iatrogenic injury.

2.16.5 Indications

1) Differentiation between hepatocellular and mechanical icterus
2) Localization of the site of obstruction (Figs. 2–5)
3) Postoperative bile duct stricture
4) Biliary atresia (relative indication)

2.16.6 Contraindications

Hepatic abscess, echinococcus cysts, acute cholangitis, bleeding disorder (prothrombin time less than 60%).

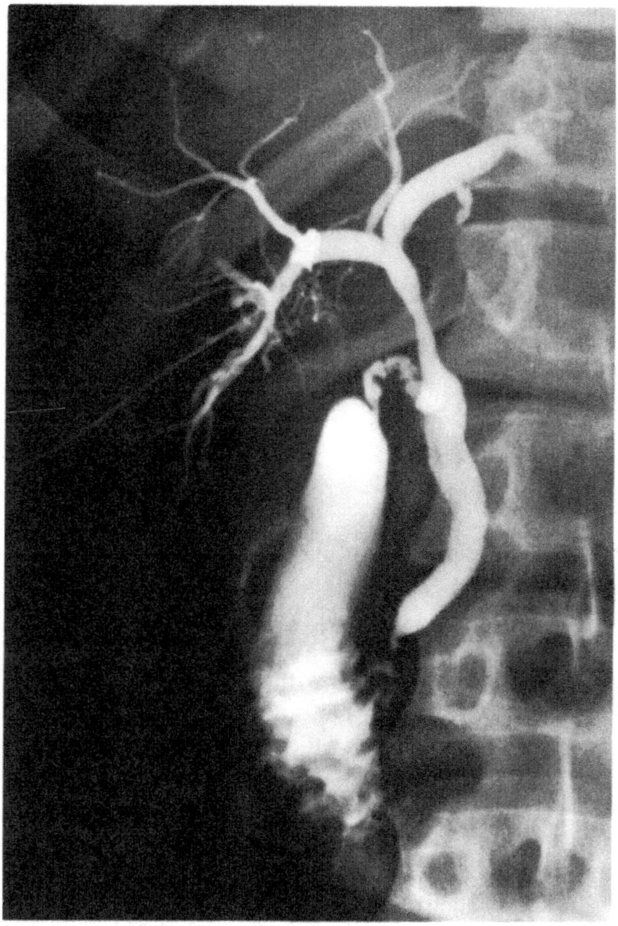

Fig. 5. Post-traumatic stenosis of the common hepatic duct after preceding hemobilia.

2.16.7 Complications

Bleeding and bile leak with bile peritonitis from the puncture tract were feared complications in the past. These complications are now avoided by use of the plastic catheter, which prevents mechanical liver injury during the inevitable respiratory excursions. The catheter can be left in place until surgical intervention for icterus due to estrahepatic biliary obstruction. Hemobilia and reactivation of acute cholangitis are extremely rare occurrences. The existence of a hemorrhagic diathesis must be excluded prior to the procedure. Inadvertent puncture of an echinococcal cyst may lead to

Table 2. Complications during 3346 percutaneous transhepatic chloangiographic procedures collected from the literature.

Bile peritonitis	27
Bleeding into peritoneal cavity	22
Shock	7
Cholangitis	6
Hemobilia	2
Blood in bile	1
Total	65 (2%)

anaphylactic shock. The complication rate is less than 2% when the above precautions are observed (Table 2).

2.16.8 Bile Duct Decompression

The *technique* of percutaneous transhepatic cholangiography may be extended in order to achieve temporary or permanent biliary drainage:

A guide wire is advanced as far as possible through the Teflon catheter which terminates in one of the bile ducts. The plastic sheath is then withdrawn and the track along the wire is enlarged with a dilator in preparation for the insertion of the drainage catheter. The latter can then usually be inserted over the guide wire without much difficulty; it is advanced into the dilated duct system until the "pig tail" tip keeps the catheter from slipping back. Finally, the external end of the catheter is sutured to the lateral wall of the thorax and is connected to a collection bag.

When the precise diagnosis has not been established already, the bile duct system should first be visualized by the "skinny needle" technique (Chiba needle). Two options exist at that point: a specially constructed thin guide wire is inserted through the Chiba needle which is then used for dilators of increasing caliber, or a second needle (catheter needle, Longdwel®) is introduced parallel to the Chiba needle (Fig. 6).

The *indications* for external bile drainage are obstructive jaundice in the inoperable patient (metastatic carcinoma of the pancreas; metastases at the porta hepatis) and preoperative decompression of the biliary system (repeat operation on the bile ducts; choledocholithiasis in high-risk patients; pancreatic resection).

Bile drainage causes a rapid decline in serum bilirubin concentration, improvement in the frequently severe pruritus, and, usually, partial relief of the dull upper abdominal pain (Köster et al, 1979).

The external catheter does create some inconveniences for the patient; meticulous skin care must be exercised and the catheter must be flushed frequently to prevent occlusion. The loss of bile acids to the outside

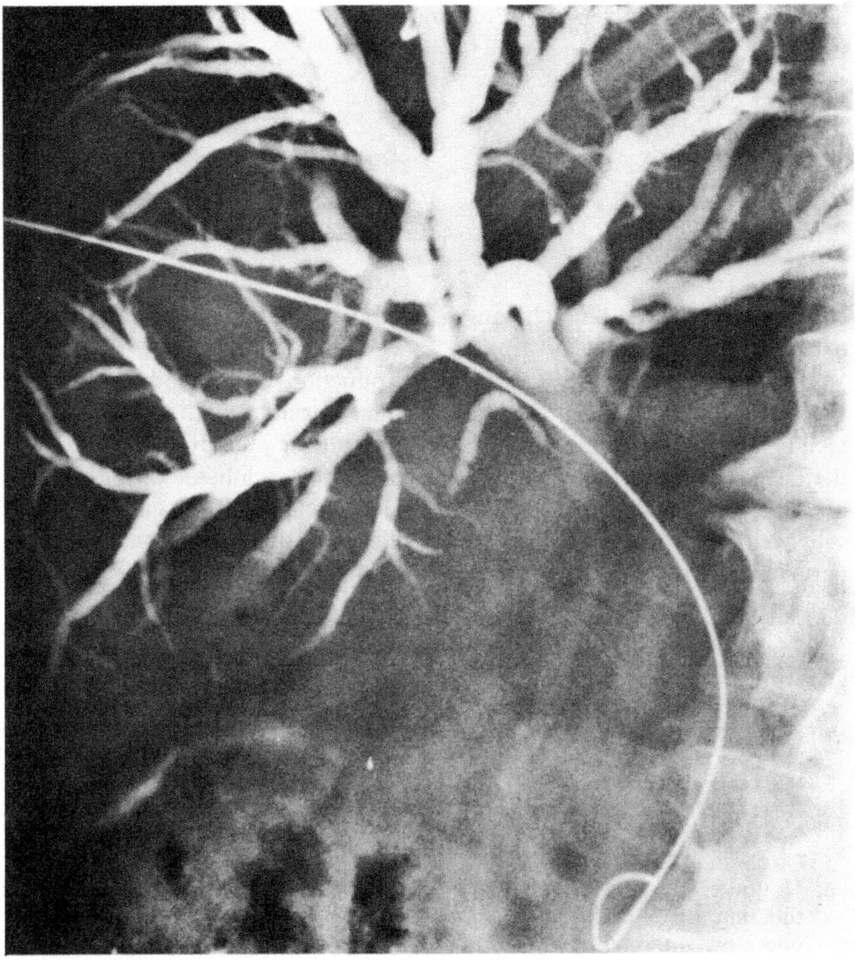

Fig. 6. Common bile duct obstruction due to chronic pancreatitis. Position of the guide wire before introduction of the drainage catheter.

has to be replaced perorally. Some of these disadvantages can be avoided by introduction of an endoprosthesis (Hoevels et al, 1978): an individually prepared length of catheter is introduced over the guide wire by use of a coaxial device. The aim is to have the tubing bridge a localized stenosis of the common hepatic duct, for instance. A smaller-caliber catheter remains in situ until successful drainage is assured.

While the experience with the endoprosthesis is still limited, the literature contains over 100 case reports of external biliary drainage. Dislodgement of the catheter by respiratory excursions is the most frequent

Table 3. Indications for external biliary drainage (n = 39). (Section of Diagnostic Radiology, University of Freiburg)

Pancreatic carcinoma	16
Bile duct carcinoma	10
Metastases at porta hepatis	5
Choledocholithiasis	3
Bile duct stricture	1
Technical failure	4

complication; ascending cholangitis and hemobilia have been observed occasionally.

In our experience (Table 3), introduction of the catheter was unsuccessful during 4 of 39 attempts at biliary drainage. The cause of these technical failures was a fibrotic liver capsule or suboptimal direction of the needle which did not permit placement of the catheter tip into a large bile duct. There were 2 complications: 1 dislocation of the catheter, and 1 subphrenic abscess following pancreatic resection performed after external drainage.

References

1. Adolph, K.: Gallengangs -und Pankreasdiagnostik. Stuttgart: Enke 1968
2. Arner, O., Hagberg, M. D., Seldinger, S. J.: Surgery. *52*, 561 (1962)
3. Bayindir, S.: Fortschr. Röntgenstr. *109*, 16 (1968)
4. Böttger, E., Burghard, A., Dittmer, F., Manegold, B.: Fortschr. Röntgenstr. *118*, 405 (1973)
5. Chudacek, Z.: Fortschr. Röntgenstr. *110*, 601 (1969)
6. Howevels, J., Lunderquist, A., Ihre, I.: Percutaneous transhepatic intubation of bile ducts for combined internal-external drainage in preoperative and palliative treatment of obstructive jaundice. Gastrointest. Radiol. *3*, 23 (1978)
7. Köster, R., Swart, B., Terwort, H.: Perkutane transhepatische Gallengangsdrainage zur präoperativen und palliativen Behandlung der Gallengangsobstruktion. Radiologe *19*, 394 (1979)
8. Rüttimann, A.: Radiol. Austria *18*, 121 (1968)
9. Wenz, W.: Radiologe *13*, 41–46 (1973)
10. Wiechel, K. L.: Acta Chir. Scand. [Suppl.] 330 (1964)

2.17

Percutaneous Transhepatic Cholangiography with the Chiba Needle

W. RÖSCH

In view of a complication rate of at least 10%, standard percutaneous transhepatic cholangiography (PTC) was limited to patients with obstructive jaundice in whom early surgery was planned [3]. In 1974, Okuda and collaborators published their first results with a variation of PTC in which a needle, 15–17 cm long and only 0.7 mm in diameter, was used, which had been developed at the Chiba University in Japan (Fig. 1). The complication rate and mortality approached zero while the biliary duct system was visualized in over 90% of all cases, with a success rate as high as 67.5% in patients with nondilated ducts.

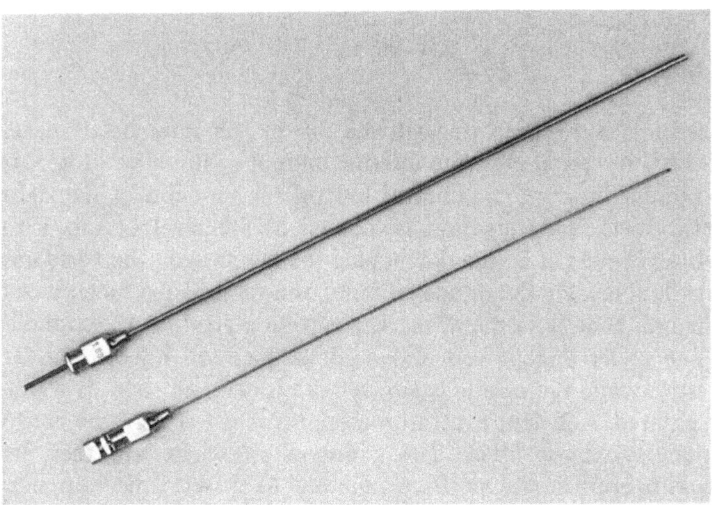

Fig. 1. Percutaneous transhepatic cholangiography: Chiba needle (below) compared to the Menghini needle (above).

2.17.1 Instruments

This form of percutaneous cholangiography requires the usual setup for local anesthesia, two Chiba needles, a 50-ml syringe with tubing about 20 cm long, and a 60% or 75% water-soluble contrast medium (Conray or Angiografin).

2.17.2 Patient Preparation

The patient is prepared as for blind liver biopsy and lies on an X-ray table. A coagulation panel should be obtained, remembering that patients with obstructive jaundice frequently are vitamin K deficient. This deficiency, if present, should have been corrected.

2.17.3 Postprocedure Care

No specific routine is needed. Minor bile spillage frequently occurs with massively dilated bile ducts, which may cause severe right upper abdominal pain. This occurrence requires potent analgesics and frequent determinations of blood pressure and pulse rate for early detection of possible bleeding. The temperature should be taken every 6 h; blood cultures should be obtained at the time of rapid temperature rise and shaking chills to rule out gram-negative bacteremia.

2.17.4 Technique

The Chiba needle is introduced through the 8th or 9th intercostal space, in the midaxillary line, parallel to the inferior margin of the liver (Fig. 2). It is advanced under fluoroscopic control toward the junction of the right and left hepatic ducts. This junction is located at the level of the 12th thoracic vertebra (Fig. 3). Landmarks include the diaphragm, the vertebral column, the air-fluid level in the duodenal bulb, or a radiopaque tube placed into the duodenum. Finally, a metal marker can be placed on the xiphoid process [6]. The stylet is removed and contrast medium injected under moderate pressure while the needle is slowly withdrawn. As soon as a bile duct has been entered, sufficient contrast material is injected until the entire intrahepatic duct system is filled. The common bile duct will then be demonstrated with appropriate position changes (Fig. 4). Injection into blood vessels is easily recognized by rapid disappearance of the contrast medium. Parenchyma injection is characterized by a slowly disappearing, rounded contrast deposit; lymphatic vessels by their convoluted course.

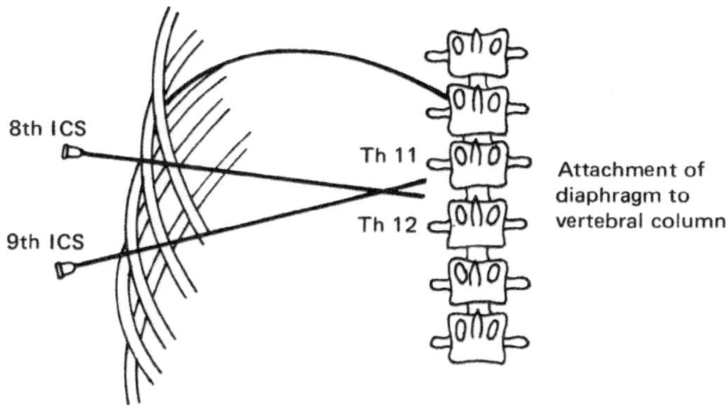

Fig. 2. Insertion through the 8th or 9th intercostal space with advancement toward the 11th to 12th thoracic vertebral body.

2.17.5 Indications

The discussion as to the relative merits and indications for percutaneous cholangiography versus endoscopic retrograde cholangiography (ERC) is still in progress [1]. PTC and ERC complement each other ideally in cases of central biliary obstruction, e.g., by cholangiocarcinoma, where the extent of the tumor can be determined precisely in both directions. In the last analysis, the expertise of the examiner should decide which of the two procedures is used first. The high diagnostic success rate in patients suspected of obstructive jaundice reported by Okuda could not be reproduced by other authors. Elias et al [2] were able to opacify dilated bile ducts with

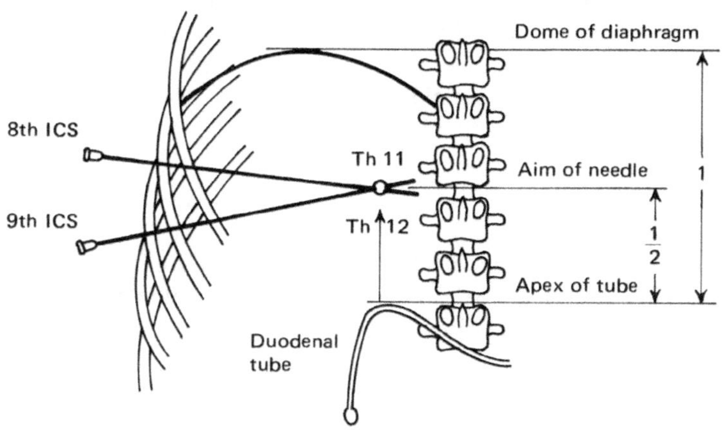

Fig. 3. Needle directed at the midpoint between diaphragm and apex of a duodenal tube.

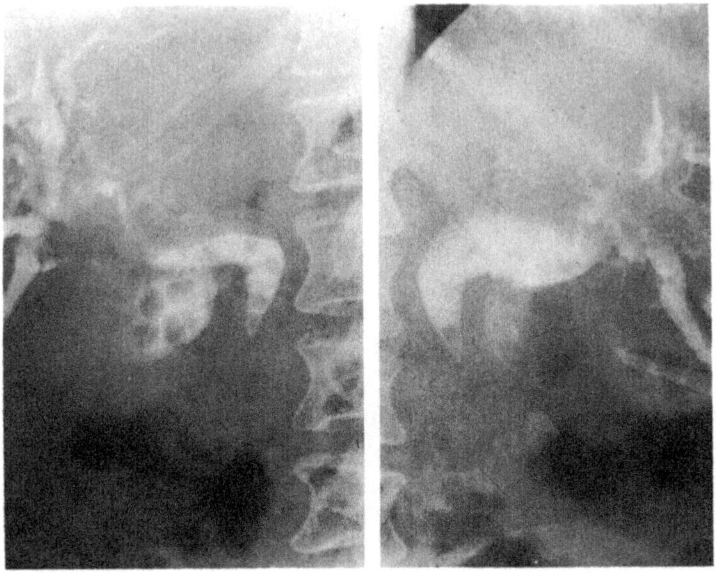

Fig. 4. Choledocholithiasis in a cirrhotic patient after Billroth II resection.

the Chiba needle in 95% of cases, but percutaneous cholangiography succeeded in only 25% of patients with intrahepatic cholestasis. However, the combined use of PCT and ERC yielded bile duct opacification in over 90% of the procedures. PTC is the only method for assessing the anastomosis in patients with choledochojejunostomy.

Our own practice is to use ERC first in patients suspected of having obstructive jaundice since this method yields additional information about the pancreas and because endoscopic sphincterotomy can be performed immediately when the common bile duct is found to be occluded by stones. On the other hand, PTC can be supplemented by long-term bile diversion in patients with inoperable obstructive jaundice.

2.17.6 Contraindications

There are essentially no contraindications to this procedure. Patients who represent unacceptable operative risks need not be excluded because the complication rate is exceedingly low.

2.17.7 Complications

Okuda presented his results at the III. European Congress for Gastrointestinal Endoscopy held in Budapest in 1976 [4]. The intrahepatic bile

Table 1. Complications with PTC and ERC (according to Okuda).

	PTC (n = 1293)	*ERC (n = 822)*
All complications	1.39%	1.06%
Bile peritonitis	0.15%	0.16%
Suspected bile leak	0.31%	
Intra-abdominal bleeding	0.08%	
Sepsis or cholangitis	0.46%	0.73%
Pneumothorax	0.15%	0.16%: acute pancreatitis
Mortality	0	

ducts were visualized in 94.3% of 1293 attempts. This rate was 100% in the presence of dilated ducts. ERC was successful in only 71.9% of 822 attempts. The complications of both procedures are shown in Table 1.

In summary, the method of choice is PTC in patients with extrahepatic bile duct obstruction; in patients with intrahepatic cholestasis, it is ERC. Both approaches should be employed with bile duct tumors to spare the patient an unnecessary explorative laparotomy when the tumor is too extensive for resection or bypass.

References

1. Conn, H. O., Redecker, A. G., Zimmon, D. S.: PTC versus ERC—an editor's dream. Gastroenterology *71*, 520 (1976)
2. Elias, E., Hamlyn, A. N., Jain, S., Long, R. G., Summerfield, J. A., Dick, R., Sherlock, S.: A randomized trial of percutaneous transhepatic cholangiography with the Chiba needle versus endoscopic retrograde cholangiography for bile duct visualization in jaundice. Gastroenterology *71*, 439 (1976)
3. Lang, E. K.: Percutaneous transhepatic cholangiography. Radiology *112*, 283 (1974)
4. Okuda, K.: Percutaneous transhepatic cholangiography with the Chiba needle. Symposium: Progress in endoscopy, radiology and ultrasonography for the differential diagnosis in disease of the liver, the bile ducts and the pancreas. IIIrd European Congress of Gastrointestinal Endoscopy, Budapest 1976
5. Okuda, K., Tanikawa, K., Emura, T., Kuratomi, S., Jinnouchi, S., Urabe, K., Sumikoshi, T., Kanda, Y., Fukuyama, Y., Musha, H., Mori, H., Shimokawa, Y., Yakushiji, F., Matsuura, Y.: Nonsurgical, percutaneous transhepatic cholangiography-diagnostic significance in medical problems of the liver. Am. J. Dig. Dis. *19*, 21 (1974)
6. Redeker, A. G., Karvountzis, G. G., Pachman, R. H., Horisawa, M.: Percutaneous transhepatic cholangiography. An improved technique. J. Am. Med. Assoc. *231*, 386 (1975)

Index

GPSR Compliance

The European Union's (EU) General Product Safety Regulation (GPSR) is a set of rules that requires consumer products to be safe and our obligations to ensure this.

If you have any concerns about our products, you can contact us on ProductSafety@springernature.com

In case Publisher is established outside the EU, the EU authorized representative is:

Springer Nature Customer Service Center GmbH
Europaplatz 3
69115 Heidelberg, Germany

Batch number: 10584442

Printed by Printforce, the Netherlands